AF699921

TABLE OF CONTENTS

Secret Key #1 - Time is Your Greatest Enemy

Pace Yourself

Wear a watch. At the beginning of the test, check the time (or start a chronometer on your watch to count the minutes), and check the time after every few questions to make sure you are "on schedule."

If you are forced to speed up, do it efficiently. Usually one or more answer choices can be eliminated without too much difficulty. Above all, don't panic. Don't speed up and just begin guessing at random choices. By pacing yourself, and continually monitoring your progress against your watch, you will always know exactly how far ahead or behind you are with your available time. If you find that you are one minute behind on the test, don't skip one question without spending any time on it, just to catch back up. Take 15 fewer seconds on the next four questions, and after four questions you'll have caught back up. Once you catch back up, you can continue working each problem at your normal pace.

Furthermore, don't dwell on the problems that you were rushed on. If a problem was taking up too much time and you made a hurried guess, it must be difficult. The difficult questions are the ones you are most likely to miss anyway, so it isn't a big loss. It is better to end with more time than you need than to run out of time.

Lastly, sometimes it is beneficial to slow down if you are constantly getting ahead of time. You are always more likely to catch a careless mistake by working more slowly than quickly, and among very high-scoring test takers (those who are likely to have lots of time left over), careless errors affect the score more than mastery of material.

Secret Key #2 - Guessing is not Guesswork

You probably know that guessing is a good idea - unlike other standardized tests, there is no penalty for getting a wrong answer. Even if you have no idea about a question, you still have a 20-25% chance of getting it right.

Most test takers do not understand the impact that proper guessing can have on their score. Unless you score extremely high, guessing will significantly contribute to your final score.

Monkeys Take the Test

What most test takers don't realize is that to insure that 20-25% chance, you have to guess randomly. If you put 20 monkeys in a room to take this test, assuming they answered once per question and behaved themselves, on average they would get 20-25% of the questions correct. Put 20 test takers in the room, and the average will be much lower among guessed questions. Why?

1. The test writers intentionally writes deceptive answer choices that "look" right. A test taker has no idea about a question, so picks the "best looking" answer, which is often wrong. The monkey has no idea what looks good and what doesn't, so will consistently be lucky about 20-25% of the time.
2. Test takers will eliminate answer choices from the guessing pool based on a hunch or intuition. Simple but correct answers often get excluded, leaving a 0% chance of being correct. The monkey has no clue, and often gets lucky with the best choice.

This is why the process of elimination endorsed by most test courses is flawed and detrimental to your performance- test takers don't guess, they make an ignorant stab in the dark that is usually worse than random.

$5 Challenge

Let me introduce one of the most valuable ideas of this course- the $5 challenge:

You only mark your "best guess" if you are willing to bet $5 on it.
You only eliminate choices from guessing if you are willing to bet $5 on it.

Why $5? Five dollars is an amount of money that is small yet not insignificant, and can really add up fast (20 questions could cost you $100). Likewise, each answer choice on one question of the test will have a small impact on your overall score, but it can really add up to a lot of points in the end.

The process of elimination IS valuable. The following shows your chance of guessing it right:

If you eliminate wrong answer choices until only this many answer choices remain:	1	2	3
Chance of getting it correct:	100%	50%	33%

However, if you accidentally eliminate the right answer or go on a hunch for an incorrect answer, your chances drop dramatically: to 0%. By guessing among all the answer choices, you are GUARANTEED to have a shot at the right answer.

That's why the $5 test is so valuable- if you give up the advantage and safety of a pure guess, it had better be worth the risk.

What we still haven't covered is how to be sure that whatever guess you make is truly random. Here's the easiest way:

Always pick the first answer choice among those remaining.

Such a technique means that you have decided, **before you see a single test question**, exactly how you are going to guess- and since the order of choices tells you nothing about which one is correct, this guessing technique is perfectly random.

This section is not meant to scare you away from making educated guesses or eliminating choices- you just need to define when a choice is worth eliminating. The $5 test, along with a pre-defined random guessing strategy, is the best way to make sure you reap all of the benefits of guessing.

Secret Key #3 - Practice Smarter, Not Harder

Many test takers delay the test preparation process because they dread the awful amounts of practice time they think necessary to succeed on the test. We have refined an effective method that will take you only a fraction of the time.

There are a number of "obstacles" in your way to succeed. Among these are answering questions, finishing in time, and mastering test-taking strategies. All must be executed on the day of the test at peak performance, or your score will suffer. The test is a mental marathon that has a large impact on your future.

Just like a marathon runner, it is important to work your way up to the full challenge. So first you just worry about questions, and then time, and finally strategy:

Success Strategy

1. Find a good source for practice tests.
2. If you are willing to make a larger time investment, consider using more than one study guide- often the different approaches of multiple authors will help you "get" difficult concepts.
3. Take a practice test with no time constraints, with all study helps "open book." Take your time with questions and focus on applying strategies.
4. Take a practice test with time constraints, with all guides "open book."
5. Take a final practice test with no open material and time limits

If you have time to take more practice tests, just repeat step 5. By gradually exposing yourself to the full rigors of the test environment, you will condition your mind to the stress of test day and maximize your success.

Secret Key #4 - Prepare, Don't Procrastinate

Let me state an obvious fact: if you take the test three times, you will get three different scores. This is due to the way you feel on test day, the level of preparedness you have, and, despite the test writers' claims to the contrary, some tests WILL be easier for you than others.

Since your future depends so much on your score, you should maximize your chances of success. In order to maximize the likelihood of success, you've got to prepare in advance. This means taking practice tests and spending time learning the information and test taking strategies you will need to succeed.

Never take the test as a "practice" test, expecting that you can just take it again if you need to. Feel free to take sample tests on your own, but when you go to take the official test, be prepared, be focused, and do your best the first time!

Secret Key #5 - Test Yourself

Everyone knows that time is money. There is no need to spend too much of your time or too little of your time preparing for the test. You should only spend as much of your precious time preparing as is necessary for you to get the score you need.

Once you have taken a practice test under real conditions of time constraints, then you will know if you are ready for the test or not.

If you have scored extremely high the first time that you take the practice test, then there is not much point in spending countless hours studying. You are already there.

Benchmark your abilities by retaking practice tests and seeing how much you have improved. Once you score high enough to guarantee success, then you are ready.

If you have scored well below where you need, then knuckle down and begin studying in earnest. Check your improvement regularly through the use of practice tests under real conditions. Above all, don't worry, panic, or give up. The key is perseverance!

Then, when you go to take the test, remain confident and remember how well you did on the practice tests. If you can score high enough on a practice test, then you can do the same on the real thing.

Top 20 Test Taking Tips

1. Carefully follow all the test registration procedures
2. Know the test directions, duration, topics, question types, how many questions
3. Setup a flexible study schedule at least 3-4 weeks before test day
4. Study during the time of day you are most alert, relaxed, and stress free
5. Maximize your learning style; visual learner use visual study aids, auditory learner use auditory study aids
6. Focus on your weakest knowledge base
7. Find a study partner to review with and help clarify questions
8. Practice, practice, practice
9. Get a good night's sleep; don't try to cram the night before the test
10. Eat a well balanced meal
11. Know the exact physical location of the testing site; drive the route to the site prior to test day
12. Bring a set of ear plugs; the testing center could be noisy
13. Wear comfortable, loose fitting, layered clothing to the testing center; prepare for it to be either cold or hot during the test
14. Bring at least 2 current forms of ID to the testing center
15. Arrive to the test early; be prepared to wait and be patient
16. Eliminate the obviously wrong answer choices, then guess the first remaining choice
17. Pace yourself; don't rush, but keep working and move on if you get stuck
18. Maintain a positive attitude even if the test is going poorly
19. Keep your first answer unless you are positive it is wrong
20. Check your work, don't make a careless mistake

General Strategies

The most important thing you can do is to ignore your fears and jump into the test immediately- do not be overwhelmed by any strange-sounding terms. You have to jump into the test like jumping into a pool- all at once is the easiest way.

Make Predictions

As you read and understand the question, try to guess what the answer will be. Remember that several of the answer choices are wrong, and once you begin reading them, your mind will immediately become cluttered with answer choices designed to throw you off. Your mind is typically the most focused immediately after you have read the question and digested its contents. If you can, try to predict what the correct answer will be. You may be surprised at what you can predict.

Quickly scan the choices and see if your prediction is in the listed answer choices. If it is, then you can be quite confident that you have the right answer. It still won't hurt to check the other answer choices, but most of the time, you've got it!

Answer the Question

It may seem obvious to only pick answer choices that answer the question, but the test writers can create some excellent answer choices that are wrong. Don't pick an answer just because it sounds right, or you believe it to be true. It MUST answer the question. Once you've made your selection, always go back and check it against the question and make sure that you didn't misread the question, and the answer choice does answer the question posed.

Benchmark

After you read the first answer choice, decide if you think it sounds correct or not. If it doesn't, move on to the next answer choice. If it does, mentally mark that answer choice. This doesn't mean that you've definitely selected it as your answer choice, it just means that it's the best you've seen thus far. Go ahead and read the next choice. If the next choice is worse than the one you've already selected, keep going to the next answer choice. If the next choice is better than the choice you've already selected, mentally mark the new answer choice as your best guess.

The first answer choice that you select becomes your standard. Every other answer choice must be benchmarked against that standard. That choice is correct until proven otherwise by another answer choice beating it out. Once you've decided that no other answer choice seems as good, do one final check to ensure that your answer choice answers the question posed.

Valid Information

Don't discount any of the information provided in the question. Every piece of information may be necessary to determine the correct answer. None of the information in the question is there to throw you off (while the answer choices will certainly have information to throw you off). If two seemingly unrelated topics are discussed, don't ignore either. You can be confident there is a relationship, or it wouldn't be included in the question, and you are probably going to have to determine what is that relationship to find the answer.

Avoid "Fact Traps"

Don't get distracted by a choice that is factually true. Your search is for the answer that answers the question. Stay focused and don't fall for an answer that is true but incorrect. Always go back to the question and make sure you're choosing an answer that actually answers the question and is not just a true statement. An answer can be factually correct, but it MUST answer the question asked. Additionally, two answers can both be seemingly correct, so be sure to read all of the answer choices, and make sure that you get the one that BEST answers the question.

Milk the Question

Some of the questions may throw you completely off. They might deal with a subject you have not been exposed to, or one that you haven't reviewed in years. While your lack of knowledge about the subject will be a hindrance, the question itself can give you many clues that will help you find the correct answer. Read the question carefully and look for clues. Watch particularly for adjectives and nouns describing difficult terms or words that you don't recognize. Regardless of if you completely understand a word or not, replacing it with a synonym either provided or one you more familiar with may help you to understand what the questions are asking. Rather than wracking your mind about specific detailed information concerning a difficult term or word, try to use mental substitutes that are easier to understand.

The Trap of Familiarity

Don't just choose a word because you recognize it. On difficult questions, you may not recognize a number of words in the answer choices. The test writers don't put "make-believe" words on the test; so don't think that just because you only recognize all the words in one answer choice means that answer choice must be correct. If you only recognize words in one answer choice, then focus on that one. Is it correct? Try your best to determine if it is correct. If it is, that is great, but if it doesn't, eliminate it. Each word and answer choice you eliminate increases your chances of getting the question correct, even if you then have to guess among the unfamiliar choices.

Eliminate Answers

Eliminate choices as soon as you realize they are wrong. But be careful! Make sure you consider all of the possible answer choices. Just because one appears right, doesn't mean that the next one won't be even better! The test writers will usually put more than one good answer choice for every question, so read all of them. Don't worry if you are stuck between two that seem right. By getting down to just two remaining possible choices, your odds are now 50/50. Rather than wasting too much time, play the odds. You are guessing, but guessing wisely, because you've been able to knock out some of the answer choices that you know are wrong. If you are eliminating choices and realize that the last answer choice you are left with is also obviously wrong, don't panic. Start over and consider each choice again. There may easily be something that you missed the first time and will realize on the second pass.

Tough Questions

If you are stumped on a problem or it appears too hard or too difficult, don't waste time. Move on! Remember though, if you can quickly check for obviously incorrect answer choices, your chances of guessing correctly are greatly improved. Before you completely give up, at least try to knock out a couple of possible answers. Eliminate what you can and then guess at the remaining answer choices before moving on.

Brainstorm

If you get stuck on a difficult question, spend a few seconds quickly brainstorming. Run through the complete list of possible answer choices. Look at each choice and ask yourself, "Could this answer the question satisfactorily?" Go through each answer choice and consider it independently of the other. By systematically going through all possibilities, you may find something that you would otherwise overlook. Remember that when you get stuck, it's important to try to keep moving.

Read Carefully

Understand the problem. Read the question and answer choices carefully. Don't miss the question because you misread the terms. You have plenty of time to read each question thoroughly and make sure you understand what is being asked. Yet a happy medium must be attained, so don't waste too much time. You must read carefully, but efficiently.

Face Value

When in doubt, use common sense. Always accept the situation in the problem at face value. Don't read too much into it. These problems will not require you to make huge leaps of logic. The test writers aren't trying to throw you off with a cheap trick. If you have to go beyond creativity and make a leap of logic in order to have an answer choice answer the question, then you should look at the other answer choices. Don't overcomplicate the problem by creating theoretical relationships or explanations that will warp time or space. These are normal problems rooted in reality. It's just that the applicable relationship or explanation may not be readily apparent and you have to figure things out. Use your common sense to interpret anything that isn't clear.

Prefixes

If you're having trouble with a word in the question or answer choices, try dissecting it. Take advantage of every clue that the word might include. Prefixes and suffixes can be a huge help. Usually they allow you to determine a basic meaning. Pre- means before, post- means after, pro - is positive, de- is negative. From these prefixes and suffixes, you can get an idea of the general meaning of the word and try to put it into context. Beware though of any traps. Just because con is the opposite of pro, doesn't necessarily mean congress is the opposite of progress!

Hedge Phrases

Watch out for critical "hedge" phrases, such as likely, may, can, will often, sometimes, often, almost, mostly, usually, generally, rarely, sometimes. Question writers insert these hedge phrases to cover every possibility. Often an answer choice will be wrong simply because it leaves no room for exception. Avoid answer choices that have definitive words like "exactly," and "always".

Switchback Words

Stay alert for "switchbacks". These are the words and phrases frequently used to alert you to shifts in thought. The most common switchback word is "but". Others include although, however, nevertheless, on the other hand, even though, while, in spite of, despite, regardless of.

New Information

Correct answer choices will rarely have completely new information included. Answer choices typically are straightforward reflections of the material asked about and will directly relate to the question. If a new piece of information is included in an answer choice that doesn't even seem to relate to the topic being asked about, then that answer choice is likely incorrect. All of the information needed to answer the question is usually provided for you, and so you should not have to make guesses that are unsupported or choose answer choices that require unknown information that cannot be reasoned on its own.

Time Management

On technical questions, don't get lost on the technical terms. Don't spend too much time on any one question. If you don't know what a term means, then since you don't have a dictionary, odds are you aren't going to get much further. You should immediately recognize terms as whether or not you know them. If you don't, work with the other clues that you have, the other answer choices and terms provided, but don't waste too much time trying to figure out a difficult term.

Contextual Clues

Look for contextual clues. An answer can be right but not correct. The contextual clues will help you find the answer that is most right and is correct. Understand the context in which a phrase or statement is made. This will help you make important distinctions.

Don't Panic

Panicking will not answer any questions for you. Therefore, it isn't helpful. When you first see the question, if your mind goes blank, take a deep breath. Force yourself to mechanically go through the steps of solving the problem and using the strategies you've learned.

Pace Yourself

Don't get clock fever. It's easy to be overwhelmed when you're looking at a page full of questions, your mind is full of random thoughts and feeling confused, and the clock is ticking down faster than you would like. Calm down and maintain the pace that you have set for yourself. As long as you are on track by monitoring your pace, you are guaranteed to have enough time for yourself. When you get to the last few minutes of the test, it may seem like you won't have enough time left, but if you only have as many questions as you should have left at that point, then you're right on track!

Answer Selection

The best way to pick an answer choice is to eliminate all of those that are wrong, until only one is left and confirm that is the correct answer. Sometimes though, an answer choice may immediately look right. Be careful! Take a second to make sure that the other choices are not equally obvious. Don't make a hasty mistake. There are only two times that you should stop before checking other answers. First is when you are positive that the answer choice you have selected is correct. Second is when time is almost out and you have to make a quick guess!

Check Your Work

Since you will probably not know every term listed and the answer to every question, it is important that you get credit for the ones that you do know. Don't miss any questions through careless mistakes. If at all possible, try to take a second to look back over your answer selection and make sure you've selected the correct answer choice and haven't made a costly careless mistake (such as marking an answer choice that you didn't mean to mark). This quick double check should more than pay for itself in caught mistakes for the time it costs.

Beware of Directly Quoted Answers

Sometimes an answer choice will repeat word for word a portion of the question or reference section. However, beware of such exact duplication – it may be a trap! More than likely, the correct choice will paraphrase or summarize a point, rather than being exactly the same wording.

Slang

Scientific sounding answers are better than slang ones. An answer choice that begins "To compare the outcomes..." is much more likely to be correct than one that begins "Because some people insisted..."

Extreme Statements

Avoid wild answers that throw out highly controversial ideas that are proclaimed as established fact. An answer choice that states the "process should used in certain situations, if..." is much more likely to be correct than one that states the "process should be discontinued completely." The first is a calm rational statement and doesn't even make a definitive, uncompromising stance, using a hedge word "if" to provide wiggle room, whereas the second choice is a radical idea and far more extreme.

Answer Choice Families

When you have two or more answer choices that are direct opposites or parallels, one of them is usually the correct answer. For instance, if one answer choice states "x increases" and another answer choice states "x decreases" or "y increases," then those two or three answer choices are very similar in construction and fall into the same family of answer choices. A family of answer choices is when two or three answer choices are very similar in construction, and yet often have a directly opposite meaning. Usually the correct answer choice will be in that family of answer choices. The "odd man out" or answer choice that doesn't seem to fit the parallel construction of the other answer choices is more likely to be incorrect.

Be Aware of the Following Hints

1. Most of the questions will focus on application of your knowledge of Neurology, Cardiology, Physiology, Pathology, Immunology, Microbiology, Dermatology, Pediatrics, Obstetrics/Gynecology, and Musculoskeletal conditions.
2. 370 questions offered given on the USMLE Step 2 test. These questions are presented in eight block formats of 46 questions within each block.
3. Each area of basic knowledge is not included with a specific block. All of the material is random. You will be required to "switch gears" between each of the above content areas.
4. Each block should be considered a separate mini-test. You have 1 hour to complete each of the eight blocks.
5. You are allowed 45-60 minutes of time for breaks. Your breaks should not be taken during a block, but following a completed mini-test and at the midpoint of testing.
6. The USMLE is offered on the computer.

Registering for the USMLE Step 2 Licensure Test

1. Contact the National Board of Medical Examiners.
2. Send in complted application with a specified testing period. You must select a testing period (3 month window). Moreover, your application must be completely process before the start date of your testing "window."
3. Receive scheduling permit, candidate idendification number, and scheduling number. You will also receive validation of your testing "window" (3 month period).
4. Contact Slyvan Prometric to set-up a testing date.
5. Take the Test

Contact Information

National Board of Medical Examiners
http://www.nbme.org

USMLE Step 2 Score Reporting

The Step 2 Committee decided to raise the three-digit score recommended to pass Step 2 CK from 182 to 184. The new minimum passing score will be applied to Step 2 CK examinations for which the first day of testing is on or after July 1, 2007

General Principles

Early cognitive development

There are four basic stages of cognitive development. Sensorimotor stage is the period from birth until approximately age 2, during which the infant develops his or her sense organs and learns that objects still exist even when they are out of the visual field. The preoperational stage typically lasts from age 2 to age 7, and is marked by the child's increasing ability to imagine the mental lives of others; in other words, to develop sympathy. The concrete operational stage generally lasts from age 7 until age 12, as the child develops a number of cognitive structures, including the rule of conservation (the understanding that an object's volume does not decrease if its shape is changed). The final stage is known as the formal operational stage and takes place after age 12. In this stage, which not every human goes through, the capacity for abstract thought (the ability to theorize rather than to rely on direct observation for knowledge) is developed.

Infancy

Infancy is defined as the period between birth and two years, in which the child undergoes significant physical, motor, vocal, cognitive, and social development. A normal baby should double its birth weight after six months and triple it after a year. During this first year, the bones should harden and calcify. Newborn infants will sleep almost constantly; by one year, the baby will be awake almost as much as it is asleep. As for motor development, it typically moves in the following sequence: head lifting, rolling, sitting, crawling, standing, and finally walking. Many infants can achieve bladder control by 18 months. The vocal ability of the child develops from consonant sounds and frontal vowels for the first ten months; by the end of the second year, however, the child may have a vocabulary of 250 words.

Puberty

At the onset of puberty, the pituitary gland begins to release the hormones that further differentiate between the sexes. Specifically, the pituitary gland releases gonadotropins, which stimulate the gonads to generate the appropriate sex hormones. As these gonadotropins do their work, the secondary sex characteristics are developed. In females, larger amounts of estrogen cause the breasts to enlarge, the hips to widen, and for fat to be deposited on the hips and buttocks. It also causes her external genitals to enlarge, and initiates the processes of ovulation and menstruation. For males, large amounts of testosterone cause the voice to deepen, the penis to become thicker and longer, muscles to grow stronger, and hair to develop in new places.

Early sexual development

There are only a few basic physiological differences between males and females. Males have the ability to make sperm and to contribute the y-chromosome that enables a female to give birth to a male. Only females are born with sex cells, menstruate, give birth, and are capable of breast-feeding. In the embryonic stage, males and females have similar sex organs. After a few weeks of development, though, the gonads differentiate into either testes or ovaries. This differentiation depends on the genetic instructions given by the sex chromosomes. If a y-chromosome is present in the embryo, it will develop into a male; if there is no y-chromosome, the embryo will develop as a female. All future differentiation will be motivated by the gonads, not the chromosomes.

Menstrual cycle

The hormones released by the female body trigger the ovaries to grow a few immature eggs. Typically, only one ovum is developed during each monthly cycle. The growth pf this hormone signals the body to produce more estrogen, which in turn produces more of the hormones responsible for menstruation. In the middle of the cycle, the egg cells are released. This is called ovulation. At this point, the body goes through many of the changes that would support a fertilized egg: the endometrium thickens and becomes richer in nourishing blood, and more estrogen and progesterone are produced. Assuming the egg remains unfertilized, the hormone levels will eventually drop and the uterine lining will be shed, resulting in some bleeding.

Perimenopause and menopause

As a woman gets older, her menstrual cycle becomes more erratic and eventually stops altogether. The period from the first irregular cycle to the last menstruation is known as perimenopause. Once a woman has not menstruated for a full year, she is said to have entered menopause. Although many women make this transition with ease, others are seriously affected. The main cause of menopausal troubles is the decline in estrogen level, which can lead to mouth and gum problems, dry or sensitive skin, hot flashes, fatigue, acne, and even hair loss. Shriveling of the clitoris, vulva, and vaginal lining may make intercourse painful. Some doctors have had success in easing women into menopause by giving them replacement hormones.

Aging

Body fat and hair -- Most individuals increase in body fat as they get older, although they also diminish in overall body size because of a reduction in muscle mass and body water content. Regular exercise, including weight training, can help to forestall these changes in body composition. Oftentimes, the higher levels of body fat in older individuals create a higher risk of disease, so it is important to monitor your weight throughout your life. The natural graying of the hair as you age is the result of the deaths of the cells that produce pigment at the base of the follicle. Individual hair shafts are thickest at age 20, and gradually shrink after that. Most individuals have hair as fine as they did as an infant once they reach the age of seventy.

Physical changes of aging -- As an individual gets older, he or she can expect his or her skin to become less resilient and more easily stretched. Of particular danger to aging skin is exposure to ultraviolet radiation from the sun. Over a long period of exposure, the skin will develop wrinkles and areas of spotty pigmentation. Human skin typically becomes drier as it ages. Also, the sweat and oil glands of the skin will naturally diminish in function with age. For most people, it becomes progressively more difficult to distinguish high-pitched and hissing noises. Indeed, hearing loss is currently ranked as the fourth most-common chronic physical disability in the United States. Even though hearing may diminish early in life, most people don't notice hearing loss until it has progressed beyond repair.

Bones and heart -- Throughout life, bones are constantly regenerating themselves in a process known as remodeling. Once a person reaches his or her mid-thirties, he or she is absorbing more old bone than he or she is creating, so bone mass decreases. This is especially problematic for women, who tend to have less dense bones than men. Bone loss for women accelerates after menopause, and about a quarter of all women will develop osteoporosis, a condition in which bones become weaker, more porous, and more vulnerable to fracture. This condition is especially common in women above the age of 60. Even though the resting heart rate stays approximately the same throughout life, the amount of blood pumped with each heart beat will decrease as a person ages. This is most apparent during exercise, as the heart takes a longer time to reach a high rate, as well as to return to its resting rate. Most of the serious heart defects that are traditionally associated with aging, such as strokes and heart attacks, are caused by arteriosclerosis and high blood pressure rather than simple deterioration from age.

Senses and teeth -- Most people in their forties will develop presbyopia, a reduced ability to focus on nearby objects. Presbyopia is caused by the slowing of the expansions and contractions of the lens. Aging individuals also are prone to cataracts, a clouding of the lens caused by natural oxidation of the eye. Most individuals who suffer from minor cataracts do not know it. It is also quite common for individuals to adjust to changes in light more slowly and to have inferior depth perception as they age. Approximately two-thirds of the taste buds in the mouth will die by the age of seventy, along with many of the smell receptors in the nose. The ability to smell is often diminished by a long-term exposure to smoke or smog. Many of the medications prescribed to elderly individuals interfere with the sense of taste. Thanks to fluorinated water and advances in dentistry, it is quite possible to have the same teeth for a lifetime. Indeed, most dental problems later in life are caused by abuse, neglect, and disease rather than aging.

Lungs and immune system -- Interestingly, the human respiratory system actually seems to become stronger with age. All of the myriad infections to which the body is exposed tend to increase the immunity, and so people tend to be somewhat resilient against colds and flu by the time they reach middle age. Also, unless an individual is out of shape or smokes, he or she should not lose any of his or her lung capacity. As for the immune system, it need not necessarily deteriorate of a person remains in shape and eats right. The only inevitable decline in the immune system that can be credited to age is a slight atrophy of the thymus gland. As people get older, they tend to be at an increased risk of cancer and infectious disease, although they are also more capable of accepting an organ transplant. Of course, being in good shape increases an individual's chances of recovering from illness at any age.

Muscles -- The muscles of the human body tend to decrease in size and strength with age, although this process can be slowed with regular exercise. The deterioration of muscle is in large part due to the body's decreased ability to synthesize protein. The lack of protein causes muscles to atrophy and lose their ability to contract. Fat and collagen tend to accumulate in the muscles as they age. Muscles also become more vulnerable to strains and cramps. Muscle strength usually declines after the age of forty, with men losing up to 20% of their strength by the age of sixty, and women often losing more. Weakening back muscles (along with deterioration of the spinal discs) account for the loss of height in aging individuals.

Brain -- When an individual reaches the age of 50, only about half as much blood will be reaching the brain as did at age 10. When a person reaches the age of 85, his or brain will have lost between 10 and 20% of its mass. Most of this weight is lost through the atrophy of nerve cells, particularly in the cerebral cortex. Although this would seem to diminish mental function, there is evidence that the brain continues to create new dendrites (that is, connections between neurons) around the nerve cells that remain. Often, individuals notice a change in their sleeping patterns as they age. In most cases, the deepest part of sleep is briefer in old age, thus accounting for the reputation of old people as light sleepers.

General principles of care

Autonomy, beneficence, nonmaleficence, disclosure -- In order to be an ethical practitioner, a doctor must respect the rights and autonomy of each patient; this entails being completely honest with each patient and allowing him or her to elect treatment. The concept of beneficence in medicine refers to the obligation of the doctor to always act in the best interest of the patient. The concept of nonmaleficence refers to the obligation of a doctor to avoid hurting a patient whenever possible. Obviously, there will be some scenarios in which the patient will elect to risk harm in order to attain some possible benefit. As for disclosure, patients are entitled to know all the details of their medical condition, including any errors that have been made by the doctor during treatment.

Conflict of interest, malpractice -- A doctor is said to have a conflict of interest when he or she has a relationship with two of the parties in a given situation. These relationships can be social, professional, or familial. For instance, if a doctor's son sells pharmaceuticals, then that doctor is said to have a conflict of interest when it comes to the prescription of non-prescription of that pharmaceutical. Doctors should try to avoid conflicts of interest as much as possible, as they tend to obscure the obligations of beneficence and nonmaleficence. As for malpractice, it can be said to occur when the doctor's dereliction of duty has directly led to damages suffered by the patient.

Confidentiality and informed consent -- All of the private information given by a patient to a doctor should be kept confidential unless the patient explicitly grants permission for the information to be disclosed elsewhere. This obligation to confidentiality can only be ignored when the patient intends to injure himself or others, is being abused by someone else, or has an infectious disease that places the general public in danger. Informed consent, meanwhile, is the patient's decision to receive a specific medical intervention. A patient can only give informed consent after learning all of the details, risks, and potential benefits of the procedure. Corollary to the idea of informed consent is the idea that the patient retains the right to change his or her mind at any time before or during the intervention.

Competence and treating minors -- In matters of consent, a doctor will often have to determine the patient's competence and decision-making capacity. A patient's competence is his or her legal capacity to be responsible for him or herself. A patient deemed incompetent is not capable of giving informed consent. A patient's decision-making capacity is his or her ability to understand the details of his or her condition as well as any proposed intervention, and to make a thoughtful decision based on this information. If a patient is a minor, then he or she is assumed to give consent in situations where he or she is unconscious and there is no available parent or guardian. Minors are not required to notify their parents regarding treatment for sexually-transmitted disease, drug or alcohol abuse, or pregnancy.

Types of death

As technology has made it possible for individuals who have in many senses died to be kept technically alive, health professionals have had to create a more complex set of definitions for death. Death is now considered as appearing in five varieties: functional, cellular, cardiac, brain, and spiritual. Functional death is when heart beat and respiration have ceased. Cellular death has occurred when the cells of the body have begun dying after the heart stops supplying them with oxygen and nutrients. Cardiac death is when the heart has stopped beating. Brain death is the termination of brain activity, in which there are no electrical impulses in the brain, and no reflexes. According to many religions, spiritual death is the moment at which the soul leaves the body.

Ethics of death

There is always a great deal of controversy surrounding individuals who lapse into a long-term coma or persistent vegetative state. There is a slight difference between the two conditions: an individual in a coma is entirely unconscious, with no memory or feelings, whereas an individual in a persistent vegetative state is awake but unaware of anything that is going on around him or her. For a long time, doctors would not allow the removal of a feeding tube, respirator, or water from an individual who was not brain-dead. In the 1970's, though, the courts allowed the removal of a ventilator from a comatose individual. The question of when or if to remove artificial means of life remains extremely contentious.

Responses to death

The great commentator on death Elisabeth Kubler-Ross has identified five stages of personal reaction to death. The first stage is denial, in which the person rejects the idea of death; this period is somewhat necessary so that the individual can overcome the initial shock of the news. The next stage is anger, in which the individual is resentful that he or she should have to die, rather than somebody else. In the next stage, the individual tries to bargain his or her way out of the predicament. In the fourth stage, depression, the individual finally begins to absorb the inevitability of his or her death, and is profoundly saddened. In the fifth and last stage, the individual accepts the inevitability of death and is neither sad nor fearful.

Preparing for death

In order to ease the process of death, may individuals compose in advance directions for their medical treatment if they should suffer a serious injury or illness. Sometimes, an individual will specify a health-care proxy, someone who is authorized to make medical decisions for them if they are unconscious or unable to act in their own behalf. Other individuals may compose what is known as a do-no-resuscitate order, in which they state that they do not want to be revived and kept alive by artificial means. An elderly or ill individual may also grant power of attorney to another person, thus giving that person the authority to make financial decisions on his or her behalf in the event of injury or illness.

Withdrawal of care and futility

A competent patient retains the right to abstain from any life-sustaining medical intervention. In all other cases, doctors are required by law to perform any interventions that can sustain life. The law does not distinguish between life-sustaining interventions that are taken away and those that a doctor fails to give in the first place. In some cases, a doctor may refuse to give further treatment on the basis of futility. Futility is established when treatment will serve no purpose, there is no reasonable point to treatment, the maximal intervention has already failed, and the intervention requested has already failed. Doctors will need to provide ample evidence for their pronouncement of futility.

Physician-assisted suicide

Despite the end of Dr. Jack Kevorkian's controversial career, there remains a great deal of argument over whether physicians should be allowed to assist the suicides of patients with terminal illness. Many doctors, with the approval of the patients' family and friends, will not pursue any extreme measures to preserve life; this is known as passive euthanasia. In other situations, though, the patient may ask that a doctor help him or her to commit suicide, if the pain of a terminal illness has become too much to bear. This practice is currently illegal in the United States, although it has been practiced for many years in the Netherlands. The American Medical Association openly states that it finds the practice of euthanasia to be unethical.

Hospice

Hospices are health-care facilities or agencies that seek to provide care for individuals in their final days. Individuals who receive hospice care may do so at a hospice facility proper, or in their own homes. In any case, the hospice strives to make the setting as comfortable and peaceful as possible. Hospice teams usually consist of nurse, physicians, chaplains, and social workers. They provide a combination of medical and emotional care not only for the fading individual, but for the friends and family at his or her bedside. Hospice facilities are able to provide the round-the-clock care that allows the loved ones of the patient to spend his or her last hours communing, rather than taking care of practical concerns.

Information bias

An information bias is one that produces a misclassification of subjects because of exposure and/or outcome. This error leads to varying data quality between groups. In a lead-time bias, the disease is diagnosed earlier, and so even though it has the same duration it appears to last for a longer period. A responder bias occurs when the patients' response to questions is affected by their knowledge that they are a part of a study. A recall bias involves any errors of memory. A measurement bias occurs when the method of gathering information distorts the data. Finally, an observer bias occurs when awareness of the hypothesis distorts the evaluation made by the observer. This last type of bias can be avoided by using a double-blind design.

Selection bias and confounding

Selection bias occurs when the relationship between an exposure and an outcome is either overestimated or underestimated because the sample that is used is not indicative of the population as a whole. Self-selection bias occurs when the sample is skewed because one type of patient is more likely to participate in a study than is another. An enrollment bias occurs when the grouping of subjects is done in a nonrandom manner. Another type of research error is confounding, which occurs when some other variable associated with an exposure also causes the outcome that is being studied and thereby skews the results. Confounding error can be minimized by correcting the research design.

Predictive value

The positive predictive value of a screening or diagnostic test is the likelihood that a patient with a positive test result actually has the disease. The positive predictive value of an exam can be calculated as the true positives divided by the total number of people who tested positive. Typically, diseases with a higher prevalence will have a higher positive predictive value. The negative predictive value of an exam, on the other hand, is the likelihood that a patient who tests negative for a disease will actually be free of it. Negative predictive value is calculated as true negatives divided by the total number of people who tested negative. A test will likely have a higher negative predictive value if the disease in question has a low prevalence.

Sensitivity and specificity

The sensitivity of a screening or diagnostic test is the likelihood that a diseased patient will have a positive test result. The sensitivity of a test can be calculated as the true positives divided by the total number of people with the disease. A test with high sensitivity may be a good screening test insofar as it can decrease the number of false negatives. The specificity of a screening or diagnostic test is the likelihood that a non-diseased person will have a negative test result. Specificity can be calculated as the true negative divided by the total number of people without the disease. Tests that have a high specificity are good at confirming the existence of a disease. In quantitative tests, however, it may be impossible to be at once highly sensitive and highly specific.

Case-control study

A case control study is one in which subjects are divided into two groups: cases (those with disease) and control (those without). Case studies attempt to determine an odds ration by obtaining information about past exposure. These kinds of studies are good in that they are usually cheap and can distinguish between multiple etiological factors. On the other hand, these studies are more likely to suffer from recall bias and survivorship bias. The latter bias occurs when patients with a particularly aggressive form of the disease die before they can be a part of the study. Also, in a case-control study prevalence, incidence, and relative risk cannot be calculated. This kind of study is especially useful in examining rare diseases and outcomes.

Incidence, prevalence, reliability and validity

The *incidence* of a disease is the number of new cases that will occur in a given at-risk population during a certain period of time.
The *prevalence* of the disease, meanwhile, is the number of cases in existence at a given time. The *reliability* of an exam is the degree to which the results can be reproduced. Inter-rater reliability is the degree to which the results of an exam vary depending on the identity of the observer. Intra-observer variability, also known as test-retest probability, is the degree to which the test results are consistent when the same person interprets the test repeatedly. The *validity* (or accuracy) of a test is the degree to which it measures what it is meant to measure. The so-called "gold standard test" is the test which has proven most reliable in measuring a particular variable.

Cross-sectional and meta-analysis

A cross-sectional study is one in which a population is surveyed at a particular time. This kind of survey is good for estimating the prevalence of a disease, but it cannot establish causal relationships for the disease since the risk factors and the prevalence of the disease are calculated at the same time. A meta-analysis, on the other hand, is a combination of the data acquired by several different studies.
Meta-analyses are good at diminishing the slight errors made by individual studies, and are often used to mitigate conflicts in research. In general, though, a meta-analysis is only as good as the studies from which the data is drawn. It is also important that the analysis be constructed properly, because errors can arise from imperfect combinations of the means and variances of different studies.

Cohort study

A cohort study is an observational study in which a group of people, known as a cohort, is tracked over time to see if they develop a certain disease. In a cohort study, data is collected in real time, which diminishes the potential for recall bias. Relative risk, incidence, and odds ratio are all easy to calculate in this kind of study, and the effects of rare exposures and multiple outcomes to an exposure can be studied. Unfortunately, the nature of the cohort study makes it impossible to examine rare diseases, and studies may be time-consuming, expensive, and plagued by selection bias and confounding variables. Most of the losses in this kind of study occur due to poor follow-up; in other words, the studies can be compromised if the researchers do not keep close track of the subjects.

AR, RR, OR, NNT

Attributable risk (AR) is the absolute difference in the incidence rate of a disease between the exposed and the unexposed populations. It is used in cohort studies.
Relative risk (RR) is defined as the likelihood of a disease developing after a patient has been exposed to a particular risk factor. Relative risk is calculated as the incidence rate of the disease in the exposed divided by the incidence rate of the disease in the unexposed.
The odds ratio (OR) is the likelihood of the disease among exposed individuals compared to unexposed individuals. It is used in both case-control and cohort studies, and is calculated by combining the exposed people with the disease and the unexposed people without disease and dividing this sum by the sum of the exposed people without the disease and the unexposed people with the disease. *The number needed to treat (NNT)* is the number of people in the general population that must be treated in order to prevent the development of disease in one person. This number is calculated as one divided by rate in the untreated group less the rate in the treated group.

RCCT

A randomized controlled clinical trial (RCCT) is a prospective study in which the subjects are randomly assigned to a treatment or control group. The randomization process diminishes bias and confounding of variables. RCCTs may be blinded (the subject does not which group he or she is in) or double-blinded (neither the subject nor the researcher knows). RCCTs are generally considered to be the best kind of study, and are especially good at establishing causal relationships. Unfortunately, preparing and administering an RCCT can be expensive and time-consuming. Also, it is simply impossible to blind some interventions. For instance, a patient will know if he or she is exercising or not. Finally, it may be unethical to give a patient a placebo instead of treatment in some situations.

Appropriate screening

Between birth and ten years of age, individuals should have the following screening measures: height and weight, blood pressure, vision, birth hemoglobinopathy screen, birth phenylalanine level, birth thyroid-stimulating hormone and T sub-4, and lead level. Between the ages of 11 and 24 years, individuals should have these screening measures: height and weight, blood pressure, Pap smear, Chlamydia and gonorrhea screening, and rubella screening and/or vaccination (females only). Individuals between the ages of 25 and 64 years should have the following screenings: height and weight, blood pressure every two years, cholesterol level every five years, Pap smear and biannual pelvic exam, fecal occult blood test, sigmoidoscopy/colonoscopy, mammography, rubella serology/vaccination (for women), and a screening for alcohol abuse and depression. Finally, patients older than 65 years should have the all of the tests appropriate for individuals between 25 and 64, as well as regular vision and hearing screenings.

Disease prevention

There are three degrees of disease prevention. First degree disease prevention entails promoting health decisions that decrease the development of a disease. Second degree prevention entails taking steps to detect a disease even when it is asymptomatic, and working to prevent its complications. Third degree prevention entails reducing the morbidity associated with the development of a disease. At present, the leading cause of death for men is prostate cancer and the leading cause of death for women is breast cancer. The second and third leading causes of death for both men and women are lung and colorectal cancer. The number of deaths attributed to lung cancer has increased since the 1950s, while the numbers of deaths caused by gastric, colorectal, and cervical cancer have all fallen.

Influenza A and Pneumococcal vaccines

The Influenza A vaccine is a trivalent killed-virus vaccine that must be administered annually. The influenza A vaccine should be administered to anyone 65 years or older; all children between 6 months and 18 years; pregnant women who are in the second or third trimester; health-care workers; and patients with cardiopulmonary disease, diabetes, hemoglobinopathies, renal dysfunction, or an immunocompromised status. Individuals with an allergy to eggs should not take the flu vaccine. Pneumococcal vaccine comes in a few types; PPV23 is the standard for adults, but children under the age of 2 years should be given PPV7. The adult vaccine is recommended for everyone over the age of 65; Native Americans and

Alaskans; and patients with chronic cardiopulmonary disease, diabetes, nephrotic syndrome, cirrhosis, asplenia, or immunosuppression.

Colorectal cancer screening

Members of the general population should begin to be screened for colorectal cancer beginning at age 50. Any polyp that is found on an endoscopy should be removed and reviewed by pathology. Any patient who has large adenomas, or more than one adenoma, should receive another colonoscopy within the next three years. Any patients with a first-degree relative with a history of colorectal cancer should begin screening at age 40. If a patient has had inflammatory bowel disease for more than 8 years, then he or she should receive surveillance with colonoscopy. If a patient has a family history of familial adenomatous polyposis, he or she should be screened using genetic analysis, and aggressive screening with colonoscopy should be initiated at age ten if the patient has the mutation. If a patient has familial adenomatous polyposis with dysplasia or persistent ulcerative colitis, then a prophylactic colectomy should be recommended.

Immunologic Disorders

Pneumonia

Diagnosis -- In order to accurately diagnose pneumonia, a doctor must perform the following tests: physical exam, complete blood count, sputum Gram stain and culture, and arterial blood gas test. In a Gram stain, the bacteria in the throat are stained with a dye called crystal violet. Pneumococci bacteria will retain the color of the crystal. Doctors may also want to perform tests for the pathogens Legionella, Chlamydia pneumoniae, and Mycoplasma. Legionella can be detected with a urine legionella sputum test, or a sputum culture. Sputum is any of the material from the lung that is brought up by coughing. Chlamydia pneumoniae can be detected with polymerase chain reaction, culture, or serologic testing. Mycoplasma can be detected with serum cold agglutinins or the serum antigen.

Introduction -- Pneumonia is an inflammation of either one or both lungs, that is usually caused by a bacterial, viral, fungal, or parasitic infection. The classic symptoms of pneumonia are fever, a cough that produces yellow-green mucus or hemoptysis (blood-stained matter), dyspnea, and pleuritic chest pain, which is caused by an inflammation of the membranes that surround the lungs. Occasionally, pneumonia will have a more gradual onset and will manifest with a dry cough, head ache, and myalgia (pain in the muscles or tissues). If a lung exam is performed, the patient will often have bronchial breath sounds or rales. Rales are sounds that can only be heard through a stethoscope and that are the result of fluid in the lungs. Patients may also display egophony or tactile fremitus.

Basic treatment for pneumonia -- Patients who have uncomplicated pneumonia can be treated with oral antibiotics. Patients who are otherwise healthy can be given macrolide, doxycycline, or fluoroquinolone. Patients who are over 65 years of age or also have COPD, renal failure, heart failure, diabetes, or liver disease should be given macrolide or fluoroquinolone. Patients with pneumonia that is so severe that it requires hospitalization should be given fluoroquinolone, extended-spectrum cephalosporin, or a beta-lactam/ beta-lactamase inhibitor. Patients who need to be admitted to the intensive care unit should be given fluoroquinolone, extended-spectrum cephalosporin, or beta-lactam/beta-lactamase inhibitors in combination with macrolide. Patients who have acquired pneumonia within a clinical environment should be given extended-spectrum cephalosporin or beta-lactam that has antopseudomonal activity.

Tuberculosis

Diagnosis -- The diagnosis of tuberculosis is frequently made with a skin test; when this test is positive the patient will receive a chest X-ray in order to determine the extent of the disease. It is very common to find tubercules, which are small bumps. The chest X-ray will also often indicate lower lobe infiltrates or apical fibronodular infiltrates that may have formed cavities. The patient should also be tested for purified protein derivative; if this test is positive, then it suggests that the patient had a prior exposure to the TB virus. It should be noted that individuals who are immunocompromised may not have a positive PPD test result even if they have been previously exposed. Their condition is called anergy, meaning that the immune system has failed to respond at all.

Introduction -- Tuberculosis is an extremely contagious bacterial infection. Most of the time, patients will develop the symptoms of tuberculosis because of a reactivation of an old infection rather than because they have just been exposed to the virus. Patients tend to be more susceptible to tuberculosis if they also have immunosuppression, alcoholism, diabetes, or some pre-existing lung condition. In recent decades, tuberculosis has become linked with the AIDS virus. In the United States, it is mandatory for tuberculosis to be treated, even if the patient cannot afford to pay for it. Some of the most common symptoms of tuberculosis are cough, weight loss, fatigue, night sweats, fever, cachexia, hypoxia, tachycardia, lymphadenopathy, and abnormal sounds during respiration.

Treatment -- There is a vaccine for tuberculosis, but it is very rarely used in the United States, in part because it is not guaranteed to work. Every case of tuberculosis has to be referred to the local health department. Patients should then receive isoniazid, pyrazinamide, rifampin, and ethambutol. Rifampin tends to turn the body fluids orange, while ethambutol is often the cause of optic neuritis. In order to prevent peripheral neuritis, an inflammation of the nerves, the patient should be given vitamin B6 at the same time as isoniazid. Rifampin and Isoniazid treatment should continue for at least six months. Also, patients whose chest X rays indicate a past exposure to tuberculosis should be given prophylactic doses of isoniazid for six months.

Acute pharyngitis

Introduction and symptoms -- Pharyngitis is simply a sore throat, or an inflammation of the pharynx. Acute pharyngitis is typically caused by viruses, but doctors should be sure to determine whether the cause happens to be Streptococcus pyogenes. Patients with streptococcal pharyngitis will present with fever, sore throat, pharyngeal erythema, and tonsillar exudates. An exudate is a fluid that seeps out of inflamed blood vessels and is deposited in nearby tissues. Other forms of pharyngitis typically present with coryza (head cold with runny nose), rhinorrhea, cough, conjunctivitis (an inflammation of the membrane that covers the surface of the eyeball), anterior stomatitis, and gastro-intestinal symptoms.

Diagnosis and treatment -- The diagnosis of acute pharyngitis can only be made through clinical evaluation, a rapid group A streptococcus antigen detection, and a throat culture. If the doctor believes that the patient may have strep throat, then he or she should begin an empiric antibiotic treatment that lasts for at least ten days. Some patients may benefit instead from amoxicillin or azithromycin. The painful symptoms of pharyngitis can be managed with fluids, rest, antipyretics, and salt-water gargles. The complications of acute pharyngitis can be suppurative (sinusitis, otitis media, mastoiditis, cervical lymphadenitis, e.g.), nonsuppurative (acute rheumatic fever, e.g.), or in the form of a peritonsillar abscess with odynophagia, lockjaw, and erythema (a redness of the skin that may be accompanied by inflammation).

Sinusitis

Symptoms -- The symptoms of sinusitis include fever, facial pain, headache, thick discolored mucus, sore throat, and a cough. A more thorough physical examination may reveal swelling or erythema (redness caused by capillary congestion) around the area in question. Acute bacterial sinusitis may manifest with a high fever, purulent nasal discharge, and leukocytosis. Leukocytosis is a condition in which the patient's level of white blood cell count is abnormally high. Patients who are being treated in the intensive care unit and have developed a fever should be checked for occult sinusitis. These symptoms occur because the mucus that has become stagnant in the sinus cavity is a perfect breeding environment for bacteria.

Introduction -- Sinusitis is an inflammation of the membrane that lines the hollow cavities around the nose. This condition can be the result of anything that impedes the airflow into and out of the sinuses. The most commonly affected areas are the maxillary sinuses. Oftentimes, the ostia (openings of the sinuses) will be blocked by swollen tissue. It is also possible for these passages to be blocked by tumors. Acute sinusitis lasts less than a month and is linked to S. pneumoniae, H. influenzae, and M catarrhalis bacteria. Chronic sinusitis lasts for more than three months and is typically caused by the obstruction of the sinus passages and minor infections. Patients with chronic sinusitis cannot effectively remove mucus from the sinus cavities.

Diagnosis and treatment -- A positive diagnosis of sinusitis can usually be made just based on clinical impression; in most cases, it will not be necessary to perform a culture. If necessary, a transillumination can be performed in which the sinus cavities will be seen to be opaque and not simply hollow. This sort of thing is only required when the symptoms of sinusitis persist for a long time. If complications are suspected, the doctor should perform a CT scan. As for treatment, the patient should be given oral amoxicillin or clavulanate for ten days. It may be beneficial for some patients to take antihistamines or nasal decongestants in order to treat the symptoms of acute sinusitis.

Meningitis

Symptoms -- Meningitis is an inflammation of the three membranes that cover the brain and the spinal cord. There are three main causes of meningitis infection: bacteria, virus, and protozoa. Patients are especially prone to developing meningitis when they have an ear infection, sinusitis, immunodeficiencies, or have had close contact with a sick person. Some people can develop meningitis because of cancer; this is known as metastasis to the meninges. Sometimes, the cause of meningitis cannot be determined. A patient with this condition will typically present with fever, malaise, headache, stiffness in the neck, and photophobia. Photophobia is an oversensitivity to light that can be extremely painful. Patient with meningitis will not be able to completely extend their lower leg perpendicular to their trunk while supine (Kernig sign).

Treatment and complications -- The particular treatment recommended for meningitis depends on the etiology of the disease. Patients should be given antibiotics as soon as possible, even before the performance of the lumbar puncture. If meningitis is caused by a viral infection, then the patient should be given supportive care and monitored closely. There are some dangerous complications associated with meningitis, including cerebral edema, subdural effusions, ventriculitis/hydrocephalus, seizures, hyponatremia, and subdural empydema. The cerebral edema will present accompanied by the absence of the oculocephalic reflex, subdural epydema will present with unstoppable seizures. Other complications of meningitis include cranial nerve palsies, coma, and death.

Diagnosis -- Individuals can be diagnosed with meningitis if they have positive Kernig and Brudzinski's signs, and if meningitis is indicated by a blood culture. A lumbar puncture may also be helpful; in this procedure, the cerebrospinal fluid is removed and submitted to a Gram stain and culture. During this procedure, the white blood cell count plus differential, red blood cell count, test for ova and parasites, and the glucose and protein levels should be obtained. A CT scan or an MRI may need to be performed in order to exclude any other diagnoses. It is common for patients with meningitis to also be suffering from leukocytosis, in which the level of white blood cells is much higher than normal.

Encephalitis

Introduction and symptoms -- Encephalitis is an inflammation of the brain, caused either by a virus, bacterium, or allergic reaction. The most common causes of encephalitis are herpes simplex virus and arboviruses, which are transmitted by mosquitoes and ticks. One of the more famous etiologies of the condition is the West Nile virus. Individuals are most susceptible to encephalitis when they are either very old or very young. The most common symptoms of encephalitis are high fever, convulsions, and coma, although individuals may also experience altered states of consciousness, lethargy, and focal neurological deficits. One particular form of the condition, known as encephalitis lethargica, causes the patient to develop a set of symptoms very similar to those associated with Parkinson's disease.

Diagnosis and treatment -- In order to diagnose encephalitis, a doctor must obtain cerebrospinal fluid; this is typically done by means of a lumbar puncture. The cerebrospinal fluid will likely demonstrate lymphocytic pleocytosis and elevated levels of protein. If the patient has red blood cells in his or her cerebrospinal fluid and does not have a history of trauma, then he or she may have encephalitis caused by the herpes simplex virus. A Gram stain of cerebrospinal fluid can be used to identify bacteria, and an acid-fast stain can be used to identify mycobacteria. Magnetic resonance imaging can be used in order to show dangerous area of abnormal tissue in the temporal lobe, especially in cases of herpes encephalitis. Patients with encephalitis cased by herpes should receive intravenous acyclovir, and patients with encephalitis due to cytomegalovirus should receive intravenous ganciclover +/- foscarnet.

HIV

Treatment -- Patients who are found to have a CD4+ count less than 350 should be given antiretroviral therapy, which attempts to fight the HIV's ability to integrate itself into the host DNA. A patient with HIV will be given two nucleoside analogs and a non-nucleoside reverse transcriptase inhibitor, or a protease inhibitor. Some protease inhibitors, which prevent proteases from dividing proteins into peptides, are so effective that they can lower the level of HIV infection such that it can no longer be detected by laboratory tests. One of the negative side effects of this treatment is lipodystrophy syndrome. The particular drug cocktail that is prescribed for a patient will depend on the patient's tolerance, drug-drug interactions, and adherence to the therapy.

Diagnosis -- The most common test for HIV is the ELISA (enzyme-linked immunosorbent assay) test, which has high sensitivity and moderate specificity. This test detects HIV by finding anti-HIV antibodies in the bloodstream. One problem with this test is that it may take as long as six months after infection for the antibodies to appear. Other tests include the Western blot, in which special proteins are separated and identified, and rapid HIV tests. After the patient has tested positive on one or more of these screening exams, he or she should be given a baseline evaluation which includes an HIV RNA PCR to test the viral load; a CD4+ cell count; a chest X ray; a Pap smear (if female); and serologoes for cytomegalovirus.

Histoplasmosis

Introduction -- Histoplasmosis is a disease caused by the fungus Histoplasma capsulatum. It can appear as acute or chronic lung disease or as progressive disseminated histoplasmosis. The most common victims of progressive disseminated histoplasmosis, which can affect a number of organs at the same time, are those who already have cancer or AIDS. Spelunking and exposure to bird or bat excrement are also risk factors for histoplasmosis. Patients with the condition may present with flu-like symptoms, including fever, weight loss, lymphadenopathy, hepatosplenomegaly, and pancytopenia. This last symptom, which is a shortage of all kinds of blood cells, is indicative of a disseminated infection.

<u>Diagnosis and treatment</u> -- A positive diagnosis of histoplasmosis is supported by a chest X-ray that indicates diffuse nodular densities, focal infiltrate, and hilar lymphadenopathy. A more sensitive test is the urine and serum polysaccharide antigen test, which also helps to determine whether treatment is helping. The chronic lung disease that often accompanies histoplasmosis is similar to tuberculosis, and will become progressively worse unless it is treated promptly. Individuals who have been diagnosed with histoplasmosis should be given amphotericin B or amphotericin B liposomal three times a day for ten days; after this, they should be given itraconazole for 12 weeks. After this, even, patients should be monitored closely and treated with antifungal medication, as the condition can come back at any time.

Candidal thrush

Candidal thrush is a yeast infection that occurs in the mucous membranes of the mouth and throat. Thrush will appear as a white plaque on the affected tissue. It is most likely to affect the elderly, young children, those with xerostemia (dry mouth) or those in an immunosuppressed state. One of the common differential diagnoses of candidal thrush is oral hairy leukoplakia, in which the individual develops white plaques on the outside borders of the tongue. This condition can usually be diagnosed based on clinical impression, though a Gram stain or potassium hydroxide test may indicates pseudohyphae or budding yeast. Candidal thrush can be remedied through hydration, dental care, and an oral nystatin suspension taken four times a day.

Pneumocystis carinii Pneumonia

Pneumocystis carinii pneumonia (PCP) is a parasitic infection of the lungs that is especially common and dangerous in very young or immunosuppressed people. The symptoms of the disorder are generally fever, shortness of breath, and bluish coloration in the extremities. If this condition is untreated, it can lead to serious lung inflammation, low levels of blood oxygen, and even fatality. This condition is often confused with tuberculosis, histoplasmosis, and coccidioidomycosis. PCP can be diagnosed after laboratory examination of the cytology of the patient's lung mucus or after a bronchoscopy specimen is treated with silver stain and immunofluourescence. Patients with this condition should be given trimethoprim-sulfamethoxazole for 21 days.

Chlamydia

<u>Introduction and symptoms</u> -- Chlamydia is a bacterial sexually transmitted disease, which is very similar to gonorrhea as far as how it is spread, its symptoms, ad its consequences over the long term. Chlamydia can infect the genital tract, the urethra, the anus, and the eyes. In women, it can wreak havoc on the Fallopian tubes, resulting in infertility, tubal pregnancy, and/ or severe pelvic infection. Perhaps unfortunately, Chlamydia is often asymptomatic; some patients, though, will present with urethritis, mucopurulent cervicitis, or pelvic

inflammatory disease. Male patients may manifest some irregular discharge or may have tender testicles, while female patients may have cervical or adnexal tenderness.

Diagnosis and treatment -- Since Chlamydia is often asymptomatic, its diagnosis depends on clinical impression. A urine test is a good way to spot the condition early and surely, and DNA probes or immunofluourescence are also accurate though they take several days. An individual diagnosed with Chlamydia should be given doxycycline at 100 mg twice a day for 7 days, or azithromycin at 1 g for one day. Every sexual partner of the afflicted individual needs to be treated as well. Chlamydia has some severe complications. Some of those who develop Chlamydia will also develop Reiter's syndrome, a systemic rheumatic disease that can cause inflammation in the eyes, mouth, heart, and skin. Other complications include epididymitis and Fitzhugh-Curtis syndrome.

Gonorrhea

Introduction and symptoms -- Gonorrhea is a bacterial sexually transmitted disease. For men, gonorrhea tends to be localized in the urethra, while in women it may infect any area of the reproductive system. The symptoms of gonorrhea are unpleasant: for men, a yellowish discharge along with an itching or burning sensation in the penis. For women, the symptoms of gonorrhea include painful and/or frequent urination, yellowish vaginal discharge, a redness or swelling of the genitals, and a burning or itching sensation around the vagina. If it is not treated effectively, gonorrhea can lead to severe pelvic infections and sterility, and in the babies of mothers with the disease it can cause eye infections. Individuals with gonorrhea may also develop swollen Bartholin's glands.

Diagnosis and treatment -- In order to diagnose gonorrhea, a swab must be taken from the infected area, whether it be the pharynx, anus, urethra, or cervix. If there is cervical discharge, a Gram stain can be taken. If the disease is disseminated, then the patient may present with monoarticular septic arthritis, rash, and/or tenosynovitis. The differential diagnosis for gonorrhea includes Chlamydia, infection of the urinary tract, vaginitis, and endometriosis. If caught early, gonorrhea can be treated effectively with antibiotics, specifically ceftriaxone injected between the muscles. Every sexual partner of the infected person needs to receive treatment as well. Patients should also be treated for Chlamydia, since there is an extremely high rate of co-infection.

Syphilis

Symptoms -- If a patient enters into the condition of second degree syphilis, then he or she is highly contagious. At this point, the rash that can develop on the palms of the hands is so contagious that it can be transmitted through extremely casual contact. If the patient enters into the third stage of syphilis, then the disease concentrates on the brain and heart, and is no longer very contagious. Nevertheless, tertiary stage syphilis can wreak havoc on the internal organs and can be fatal in some cases. Some individuals will be latent carriers of syphilis. Early latent individuals will have no symptoms but a positive serology, while late latent individuals will have no symptoms, either a positive or negative serology, and will have had the infection for at least a year.

Introduction -- Syphilis is a sexually transmitted disease caused by Treponema pallidum, a tiny organism otherwise known as a spirochete. This tubular organism buries itself in the mucous membranes of the mouth or genitals, and there produces the painful ulcers known as chancres. Patients with first degree syphilis will present with chancres that are not yet the source of any pain. Second degree syphilis begins between four and eight weeks after the infection for about a quarter of all those infected; during this period, the patient may present with hair loss, a sore throat, and white patches on the mouth or genitals. If the patient has an especially vicious case of syphilis, then he or she may present with a mucous patch or condylomata lata, warts growing around his or her anus.

Diagnosis and treatment -- Some of the common identifiers of third-degree syphilis are granulatous gummas, tabes dorsalis (the steady degeneration of the spinal cord), meningitis, and the Argyll Robertson pupil (in which the pupil can constrict but does not react to light). Syphilis can be diagnosed after dark-field microscopy indicates motile spirochetes and the rapid plasma reagin test developed by the Venereal Disease Research Laboratory is positive. This latter exam may occasionally give false positive if the individual is a drug user, has rheumatic fever, has another virus, or has leprosy. As for treatment, first degree syphilis can be treated with benzathine penicillin injected between the muscles, while a latent infection can be treated with penicillin once a week for three weeks. If a patient has developed the neurological symptoms of third degree syphilis, then he or she should be given intravenous penicillin.

Urinary tract infections

Introduction and symptoms -- A urinary tract infection is found in the kidney, ureter, bladder, or urethra. This condition affects women more often than men. Some of the risk factors for urinary tract infections are catheters, anatomic irregularities (as for instance vesicoureteral reflux or benign prostatic hyperplasia), a history of urinary tract infection, diabetes, recent use of antibiotics, pregnancy, and conditions of immunosuppression. Some UTIs are asymptomatic, while others may manifest with dysuria, suprapubic pain, frequency of urination, and sometimes hematuria. A differential diagnosis for urinary tract infection may include vaginitis, sexually transmitted diseases, prostatitis, or acute urethral syndrome.

Diagnosis and treatment -- A urinary tract infection can be diagnosed after a urine dipstick or urinalysis reveals an elevated level of the leukocyte esterase, elevated nitrates (which indicate bacteria), and elevated urine pH. A microscopic analysis may indicate pyuria (pus in the urine, signifying inflammation) and bacteriuria. The gold standard test for urinary tract infection is a urine culture that indicates levels greater than 10 to the fifth power CFU/mL. If the patient is a healthy young female, she may be treated with oral TMP-SMX or fluoroquinolone for three days. Patients who are considered to be at a greater risk of severe infection can get he same medication, but over the course of a week or ten days. Those patients with urosepsis require immediate hospitalization and intravenous antibiotics.

Pyelonephritis

Pyelonephritis is a bacterial infection of the kidneys, usually caused by the upward movement of bacteria from the bladder into the ureters, where they go on to infect the kidneys. Pyelonephritis is almost always caused by the same pathogen that causes cystitis, and the two conditions have the same risk factors. The common symptoms of pyelonephritis include flank pain, fever, chills, malodorous urine, frequent urination, and general malaise. The patient will often have tenderness in the kidney if it is gently tapped with a fist. The diagnosis of pyelonephritis is similar to that of cystitis, with the exception that urinalysis and culture are accompanied by white blood cell casts. A complete blood count will often indicate leukocytosis. Patients can be treated with fluoroquinolone or another antibiotic.

Sepsis

Introduction and symptoms -- Sepsis is the contamination of the blood or tissues of the body with bacteria or infectious organisms. Sepsis, then, is a systemic inflammatory response syndrome that has a documented infection. The symptoms of sepsis may be like those of other systemic illness: fever, chills, malaise, low blood pressure, and alterations in mental state. Sepsis can be fatal. If a patient enters septic shock, then he or she may develop hypotension or organ dysfunction caused by inadequate perfusion. Typically, patients with sepsis will have a sudden onset of fever and chills, tachycardia, and tachypnea. Septic shock usually presents as warm skin and extremities, though the body may be cool if there are other complications, as for instance congestive heart failure.

Diagnosis and treatment -- Since sepsis usually arises out of some other condition, its diagnosis is dependent on clinical impression. The patient will likely have leukocytosis or leucopenia with an increased number of bands. Half of all cases of sepsis will be accompanied by thrombocytopenia, and many cases will manifest elevated levels of creatine or LFTs. A patient with sepsis may test positive for bacteria in the blood, urinem or sputum if a culture is performed. Doctors should make a coagulation study and consider a disseminated intravascular coagulation panel. Patients with severe sepsis may need to be admitted to the intensive care unit. Otherwise, sepsis should be treated by focusing on the underlying cause. The overarching concern of a doctor in the treatment of sepsis is to maintain the blood pressure and flow to the internal organs.

Osteomyelitis

Introduction and symptoms -- Osteomyelitis is an inflammation of the bone that is caused by an infection, as for instance salmonella or staphylococcus. It usually comes from a soft tissue infection, though in children and intravenous drug users it can often be the result of hematogenous seeding. It is possible for both the bone and the bone marrow to become infected. The symptoms of osteomyelitis include severe pain and muscle spasms in the areas that have been infected, as well as fever. This condition is commonly linked with diabetes, intravenous drug abuse, and peripheral vascular disease. It is rare but worth mentioning that some patients will present with fever, chills, and purulent drainage/limited motion in the afflicted area.

Diagnosis and treatment -- A positive diagnosis of osteomyelitis can be made after lab tests indicate elevated C-reactive protein, erythrocyte sedimentation rate, and white blood cell count. Although X-rays of the affected area may be negative at first, they may indicate an inflammation of the periosteum (the membrane covering the bone) within two weeks time. The gold standard test for osteomyelitis is a bone aspiration accompanied by Gram stain and culture. The treatment for the condition is a surgical debridement of the dead/infected bone. The patient should then be given intravenous antibiotics for 4-6 weeks. Some of the dangerous complications of osteomyelitis include sepsis, septic arthritis, and even squamous cell carcinoma.

Lyme disease

Introduction and symptoms -- Lyme disease is caused by the bacterium Borrelia burgdorferi, which is carried by the deer tick. This condition is almost always manifested during the summertime. It is especially common in the Northeast, northern Midwest, and Pacific coast. The infection, once it enters the body, can infect a number of tissues and cause a variety of symptoms. There are three basic phases of Lyme disease. First degree Lyme disease entails inflammation of the area of the bite; second degree Lyme disease entails migratory polyarthropathies, meningitis, conduction abnormalities possibly including third-degree heart block; third-degree Lyme disease entails arthritis and subacute encephalitis.

Diagnosis and treatment -- The diagnosis of Lyme disease depends on the accurate identification of the erythema migrans, the classic rash reaction in which the skin surrounding the bite develops a red, unraised ring. The patient can then be given ELISA and Western blot tests; the ELISA test, it should be noted, only can be used to determine whether the patient has been exposed, and not whether he or she has been infected. If the disease is caught early, the patient can be given doxycycline; if it is caught late, then he or she can be given ceftriaxone. It may be necessary to administer empiric antibiotics to those patients who develop arthralgias (joint pain), rash, or were bitten by the tick in an area where Lyme disease is common.

Neutropenic fever

A neutropenic fever occurs when an individual has a significant decrease in the number of neutrophils in his or her body and subsequently develops a fever greater than 38.3 degrees Celsius for more than an hour. This condition is fairly common in cancer patients who are enduring chemotherapy. Patients who are suspected of neutropenic fever should be given a thorough physical examination; however, because of the possibility that the patient has a diminished number of white blood cells, a rectal examination should not be performed. It may also be helpful to diagnosis to perform a complete blood count. Patients who are given a positive diagnosis of neutropenic fever should be given antibiotics for 72 hours; if the symptoms persist, antifungals should be administered.

Rocky Mountain spotted fever

Rocky Mountain spotted fever is an acute febrile disease that is caused by Rickettsia ricketsii and is transmitted by hard-shelled ticks. This organism attacks the layer of cells that line the closed internal parts of the body, and can cause vasculitis, or inflammation, of the small vessels. Patients with Rocky Mountain spotted fever will frequently present with headache, fever, rash, and malaise. The rash associated with this condition begins on the extremities but quickly spreads toward the central regions of the body. In order to diagnose this condition, a biopsy of the patient's rash should be submitted to indirect immunofluourescence. The appropriate medication for Rocky Mountain spotted fever is doxycylcine or chloramphenicol.

Infective endocarditis

Introduction -- Infective endocarditis is an infection of the endocardium, the lining of the internal surface of the heart chambers. This condition is usually preceded by some bacterial or other infectious cause. It is extremely dangerous, as it can affect the valves of the heart. Individuals are considered to be at a greater risk of infective endocarditis if they have prosthetic heart valves, use intravenous drugs, suffer from immunosuppression, or have rheumatic, valvular, or congenital heart disease. The following bacteria are associated with the development of infective endocarditis: S. aureus (especially in IV drug users), Staphylococcus (especially for those with prosthetic heart valves), Streptococcus bovis (especially among those with a preexisting gastrointestinal malignancy), and Viridans streptococci.

Symptoms, diagnosis and treatment -- Patients with infective endocarditis will present with weakness, dyspnea, chills, anorexia, and skin lesions. A physical exam will indicate heart murmur, and may discover Osler's nodes (small and tender nodules on the palms of the hands and soles of the feet), Janeway lesions, splinter hemorrhages, and Roth's spots (hemorrhages of the retina). The diagnosis of infective endocarditis depends on the Duke criteria: major endocarditis must be supported by two positive blood cultures and evidence of endocardial involvement, while minor endocarditis can be supported by the presence of risk factors, a fever, characteristic vascular and immunologic phenomena, and substantial microbiological evidence. Infective endocarditis can be treated with empiric antibiotics, for example vancomycin.

Coccidioidomycosis

Coccidioidomycosis is a fungal disease that comes from spores that live in the desert sands of the American Southwest. The symptoms of this condition include fever, cough, muscle pain, and occasionally severe lung disease. The infection needs to incubate for between one and four weeks after exposure. A diagnosis of the condition can be made after a serology test indicates elevated levels of precipitin antibodies within two weeks of exposure; these elevated levels will cease after a couple of months. A doctor may also want to take cultures of the joint aspirate, wound exudate, or sputum. A chest X-ray may indicate infiltrates, nodules, or pleural effusion. A patient diagnosed with coccidioidomycosis should be given amphotericin B or itraconazole.

Anthrax

Anthrax is a highly contagious disease that most commonly affects animals, but is occasionally transmitted to humans through incidental contact with animals or their products. Anthrax is also a popular feature of biological weapons. The symptoms of anthrax can be either gastrointestinal (dysphagia, abdominal pain, and bloody diarrhea), cutaneous (lesions, lymphadenopathy, eventual black eschars), or inhalational (fever, dyspnea, hypotension, and symptoms of pneumonia). The diagnosis of anthrax can be made after a Gram stain and aerobic culture of the exudate from the ulcer indicates short chains of the anthrax bacilli. The treatment for anthrax includes antibiotics like penicillin, tetracycline, erythromycin, and ciprofloxin.

Otitis externa

Otitis externa, otherwise known as swimmer's ear, is simply an infection of the outer auditory canal. It is caused either by Pseudomonas or enterobacteriacae bacteria. Patients suffering from otitis externa may present with pain, pruritus, or purulent discharge. A more comprehensive examination of the ear will reveal that the pinna (the part of the ear that extends perpendicular to the head) will have moved, and the patient will have an erythematous and edematous ear canal. The diagnosis of otitis externa is usually made on clinical impression, although the precise fungal cause of the infection can be determined by a Gram stain and culture. The most immediate treatment for the condition is a program of neomycin or polymyxin eardrops; patients with severe disease may require systemic antibiotics.

Blood Diseases

Idiopathic thrombocytopenic pupura

Idiopathic thrombocytopenic pupura (ITP) is am autoimmune platelet disorder that causes the IgG autoantibody to bind to platelets and lead to lysis by splenic macrophages. When an individual has ITP accompanied by autoimmune hemolytic anemia, it is called Evans' syndrome. Individuals, usually females, are most likely to manifest ITP during between the ages of 20 and 50. When ITP occurs in pediatric patients, it typically does so with an acute onset preceded by some viral illness. In adults, on the other hand, ITP inset usually follows a viral infection, and is occasionally brought on by sulfa drugs. ITP has no systemic symptoms, and typically does not cause fever. When bleeding is in the mucosa or skin, it may include epistaxis, oral bleeding, menorrhea, purpura, or petechiae.

In cases of supposed idiopathic thrombocytopenic pupura where splenomegaly also exists, doctors should consider an alternative diagnosis. In general, ITP is diagnosed after everything else has been ruled out. A complete blood count should show thrombocytopenia, and occasionally will also show anemia. The patient will likely demonstrate a positive platelet-associated IgG test, and a peripheral blood smear will often indicate megathrombocytes without schistocytes. Treatment for pediatric cases of ITP should take into account that the disease is largely self-limited, and will usually resolve in between four and six weeks. Adults may require only observation for mild ITP, but patients with a severe hemorrhage or thrombocytopenia should receive intravenous gamma globulin anti-Rho (D). In cases of uncontrollable bleeding, platelets should be administered.

Von Willebrand's disease

Von Willebrand's disease is the hereditary bleeding disorder that affects the most people. It is caused by deficient or abnormal amounts of von Willebrand's factor, which helps to stabilize factor VIII and can augment the aggregation or attachment of platelets to injured vascular endothelium. This condition typically presents with mild bleeding, which is usually mucosal but can also be gastro-intestinal. These symptoms will tend to increase if the patient takes aspirin. A positive diagnosis of von Willebrand's disease can be made after lab tests indicate the patient has diminished levels of activated factor VIII, as well as low levels of von Willebrand's factor. Also, the patient will demonstrate excessive bleeding time. Treatment for von Willebrand's disease involves fresh frozen plasma for major bleeding, and DDAVP for mild cases.

Hemophilias

Hemophilias are x-linked recessive coagulopathies that are caused by diminished factor VIII or factor IX. Diminished factor VIII leads to hemophilia A, while diminished factor IX leads to hemophilia B. The degree to which factor VIII or IX is diminished will determine the severity of bleeding. If the bleeding is mild, for instance, then it will only occur after a major trauma or surgery. If, on the other hand, bleeding is moderate, then the patient will bleed after mild trauma or surgery. Bleeding is classified as severe when it begins spontaneously. A diagnosis of hemophilia can be made after a prolonged examination of activated partial thromboplastin time. Also, of course, hemophilia can be diagnosed when the patient is found to have diminished levels of factor VIII or IX. In order to treat hemophilia, a factor VIII or IX concentrate should be given during bleeding and as a preventive before surgery.

Hypercoagulable state

Introduction -- Hypercoagulable states are associated with an elevated risk of thromboembolic disease, including deep venous thrombosis, pulmonary embolus, and cerebrovascular accidents. The inherited causes of hypercoagulable states include: factor V Leiden; protein C or S deficiency; antithrombin III deficiency; homocystinemia; fibrinolysis defects; and prothrombin gene mutation. The acquired causes of hypercoagulable states include: cancer; myocardial infarction; prolonged bed rest or immobilization; pregnancy; tissue damage; hyperlipidemia; vasculitis; multiple myeloma; lupus anticoagulant; nephritic syndrome; smoking; warfarin; myeloproliferative disorders; paroxysmal nocturnal hemoglobinuria; heparin-induced thrombocytopenia or thrombosis; and TTP.

Symptoms -- Individuals with a congenital hypercoagulable state often present with venous thrombosis or recurrent thromboembolism; typically, these patients will either be in late adolescence or early adulthood. For the majority of patients, it is not necessary to do an entire lab workup for hypercoagulable state after the first appearance of deep venous thrombosis. However, patients who develop the condition in an unusual location, as for instance the hepatic, mesenteric, and splenic venous beds, should be monitored, as should those who have recurrent episodes of deep venous thrombosis. If the patient has an arterial thrombosis, this may appear first as a large-vessel occlusion, like a stroke or myocardial infarction, or as a microvascular problem, like erythromelalgia.

Diagnosis and treatment -- In order to determine the nature of a patient's hypercoagulable disorder, the doctor should look for a history of miscarriages. Doctors can suspect pulmonary embolism in patients that have a rapid onset of tachypnea, tachycardia, hypoxia, hypocapnia, and an A-a gradient without the presence of another possible explanation. An inherited hypercoagulable state can be diagnosed after lab tests on factor V Leiden, prothrombin gene mutation, antithrombin III, protein S and protein C assays. The diagnosis of acquired hypercoagualable state is made by looking for an underlying cause. If the patient should require surgery, he or she should be given a small amount of heparin, like 5000 U q 8-12 h) in order to decrease thrombosis before the operation. As for congenital biochemical defects, they can often be treated effectively with warfarin.

Leukemia

Leukemia is a malignant proliferation of hematopoietic cells. The type of leukemia diagnosed is based on the cellular origin and on the degree of differentiation between the neoplastic cells. There are four basic subtypes of leukemia: acute leukemias are proliferations of very slightly differentiated blast cells; chronic leukemias are proliferations of more mature and differentiated cells; lymphocytic leukemias are neoplasms of lymphoid cells; and myelogenous leukemias are neoplasms of myeloid cells. The signs of leukemia can be more easily remembered using the mnemonic LEUKEMIA: light skin; energy decrease; underweight; kidney failure; excess heat; mottled skin; infections; and anemia.

Acute lymphocytic leukemia

Introduction and symptoms -- Acute lymphocytic leukemia (ALL) is a form of the disease that is especially common in children and is more likely to occur in Caucasians than African-Americans. This form of leukemia manifests in an acute onset of symptoms, usually within a few weeks of diagnosis. Patients suffering from acute lymphocytic leukemia will complain of malaise, fever, lethargy, and weight loss. It is also quite common to discover bone pain, infection, and hemorrhage. A more thorough physical examination will often reveal lymphadenopathy and hepatosplenomegaly. When a complete blood count is made, it will indicate a depression of bone marrow elements, as in anemia or thrombocytopenia, and either a high or a low leukocyte count.

Diagnosis and treatment -- A positive diagnosis of acute lymphocytic leukemia can be made after lab tests indicate high levels of uric acid and lactate dehydrogenase. A marrow biopsy will reveal elevated blasts with positive PAS, TdT, and CALLA. Cytogenetics can also be sued to make a diagnosis of acute lymphocytic leukemia. Between 25 and 30% of patients will have the so-called Philadelphia chromosome, technically known as t(9;22); these patients have a lower chance of recovery than do others. The majority of cases of acute lymphocytic leukemia have a B-cell lineage and express CD10 (CALLA antigen) and CD19+/-CD20. Some 15 to 20% of the instances of acute lymphocytic leukemia are of T-cell lineage and express CD2, CD5, and CD7.

It is often useful when trying to make a diagnosis of acute lymphocytic leukemia to perform a chest CT scan in order to rule out the possibility of mediastinal involvement. A lumbar puncture is often performed in order to exclude the possibility of leptomeningeal involvement. A head CT scan may be performed in order to rule out the possibility of parenchymal brain involvement. The treatment for acute lymphocytic leukemia always includes chemotherapy, during which vincristine, prednisone, daunorubicin, L-asparaginase, and cyclophosphamide are often used. Less than one percent of pediatric patients fail to achieve full remission with chemotherapy, and four out of five will survive over the long-term with leukemia. The prognosis for adult patients is not quite so good. Those patients who are found to have the Philadelphia chromosome often will require bone marrow transplants.

Acute myelogenous leukemia

Introduction -- Acute myelogenous leukemia can be divided into eight basic subtypes, numbered M0 through M7. The subtype is based on neoplastic cell type and cytogenetics. This form of leukemia most commonly affects adults, and the incidence level tends to increase with age. Patients will typically present with fatigue, hemorrhage, and bruising, and it is common also to observe the symptoms of bone marrow failure, as for instance anemia, thrombocytopenia, and neutropenia. A small number of patients, less than a quarter, will present with splenomegaly, hepatomegaly, and lymphadenopathy. Disseminated intravascular coagulation is often associated with subtype M3, while gingival hyperplasia is often associated with subtype M5.

Symptoms -- Oftentimes, patients who have a high white blood cell count will present with the symptoms of leukostasis, meaning that there is an accumulation of thick leukemic blast in the tissue microvasculature. The symptoms of leukostasis can include confusion, somnolence, stupor, coma, exertional dyspnea, respiratory distress, disseminated intravascular coagulation, retinal hemorrhage myocardial infarction, acute limb ischemia, and renal vein thrombosis. A positive diagnosis of acute myelogenous leukemia can be made after a complete blood count with differential indicates varying levels of anemia and thrombocytopenia. The white blood cell count for a patient with this condition may be high, normal, or low. A disseminated intravascular coagulation panel will indicate elevated prothrombin time, diminished levels of fibrinogen, and positive fibrin split products.

Diagnosis and treatment -- As part of making a diagnosis of acute myelogenous leukemia, a doctor should have a peripheral blood smear and a marrow biopsy that indicate elevated blast levels, Auer rods, and positive Sudan black and myeloperoxide stains. As for cytogenics, those patients with t(8;21), t(15;17), and inv(16)(p13;q22) are likely to have a favorable outcome, while monosomy 5 and 7 and complex abnormalities are less likely to have a positive outcome. Individuals with acute myelogenous leukemia type M3 with t(15;17) have a translocation involving the retinoic acid receptor alpha and promyelotic leukemia, or PML genes. Patients with this form of leukemia receive chemotherapy, including cytarabine accompanied by anthracycline. Those patients with negative cytogenetics or who do not enter into remission should receive stem cell transplantation. Type M3 should be treated with all-trans-retinoic acid. It may be necessary to perform leukpheresis or immediate chemotherapy on those patients with a high white blood cell count.

Chronic lymphocytic leukemia

Introduction and symptoms -- Chronic lymphocytic leukemia is a clonal malignancy of B and T lymphocytes. The B lymphocytes will make up more than 98% of the malignancy. Chronic lymphocytic leukemia has a very slow progression; there will be a slow accumulation of durable lymphocytes that are immunocompetent. The median age for the onset of chronic lymphocytic leukemia is 65. Most cases of CLL will be asymptomatic, although some victims may complain of fatigue, lymphadenopathy, and splenomegaly. It is more common for infections to occur after neutropenia or hypogammaglobulinemia. In the later stages of the disease, a patient may develop fever, night sweats, and weight loss.

Diagnosis and treatment -- A positive diagnosis of chronic lymphocytic leukemia requires a confluence of measures. A complete blood count will often indicate an incidental finding of isolated lymphocytosis, in which the lymphocyte count is greater than 5000. The whole blood count will often be greater than 20,000 microliters and may be greater than 100,000 microliters. On the other hand, it is common for individuals with chronic lymphocytic leukemia to have a normal hematocrit and platelet count. If a peripheral blood smear is taken, this will usually indicate minute, mature cells with condensed nuclear chromatin along with smudge cells. Smudge cells are leukocytes that have been damaged during smear preparation because of cell fragility.

A diagnosis of chronic lymphocytic leukemia is suggested when the patient's bone marrow has been penetrated by small lymphocytes. A flow cytometry will indicate a coexpression of CD19 and CD5. About half of the cases of chronic lymphocytic leukemia will have hypogammaglobulinemia. If cases of indolent chronic lymphocytic leukemia are diagnosed early, then only supportive therapy is required. Patients will be more benefited by chemotherapy when they demonstrate progressive fatigue, symptomatic lymphadenopathy, or anemia/thrombocytopenia. Chemotherapy may include fludarabine (unless there is autoimmune hemolytic anemia), chlorambucil (better for older patients), and rituximab (can be used to treat autoimmune hemolytic anemia). Patients with associated autoimmune hemolytic anemia and immune thrombocytopenia are treated effectively with prednisone and splenectomy.

Chronic myelogenous leukemia

Introduction and symptoms -- Chronic myelogenous leukemia is a clonal stem cell disorder in which there is a proliferation of myeloid cells at every possible level of differentiation. The median age for the onset of this form of leukemia is 42 years. Patients will typically present with fatigue, night sweats, and a slight fever. A physical examination will often indicate abdominal fullness caused by splenomegaly. In the chronic phase of chronic myelogenous leukemia, the patient will have an elevated white blood cell count as well as enlarged liver and spleen. In the accelerated phase of the disease, the patient will have a diminished level of red blood cells and platelets, bone pain, fever, night sweats, and weight loss. In the blast phase of the disease, the patient's peripheral blood and marrow will be infiltrated by proliferating leukemic blast cells.

Diagnosis -- Patients with chronic myelogenous leukemia will have a significantly high level of white blood cells; indeed, the median white blood cell count at the time of diagnosis is 150,000 microliters. It is also possible for basophilia and eosinophilia to be present. Hematocrit will be normal, and the platelet count will either be normal or slightly elevated. Patients in the accelerated or blast phases may have anemia or thrombocytopenia. A peripheral blood smear will indicate that the myeloid series is shifted to the left with mature forms dominating. Almost nine out of ten patients will have the Philadelphia chromosome, t(9;22), which can lead to bcr-abl gene. Also, patients with chronic myelogenous leukemia will have diminished levels of leukocyte alkaline phosphatase.

Treatment -- An examination of the bone marrow of a patient with chronic myelogenous leukemia will frequently reveal that it us hypercellular with myelopoiesis shifted to the left. The blast phase of this form of leukemia can be diagnosed when the blasts make up more than 20% of the bone marrow. Chemotherapy is the most common kind of treatment for CML. The drug imatinib mesylate, otherwise known as Gleevec, can limit the activity of tyrosine kinase of the bcr-abl oncogene. One drug that has great results but occasionally severe side effects is interferon-alpha. Patients who cannot withstand any other treatments can be given hydroxyurea. Patients less than 60 years of age can be given an allogeneic bone marrow transplant. One of the dangerous complications of CML is leukostasis clinical syndrome.

Non-Hodgkin's lymphomas

Non-Hodgkin's lymphomas are basically just a monoclonal proliferation of B or T lymphocytes. Patients will be at special risk of developing Non-Hodgkin's lymphomas when they have Epstein-Barr virus or HIV. These are the largest group of hematologic neoplasms, and will typically have a noncontinuous lymph node spread. Patients will often present with painless adenpathy and B symptoms, which include low-grade fever, night sweats, and slight weight loss. A more thorough physical examination will frequently reveal systemic adenopathy or hepatosplenomegaly. A biopsy must be performed in order to make the diagnosis; chest X-rays, full-body CT scans, and a bone marrow biopsy and lumbar puncture may be helpful. Treatment for Non-Hodgkin's lymphomas typically includes radiation and chemotherapy.

Hodgkin's lymphomas

Hodgkin's lymphomas are lymph malignancies that arise out of proliferating germinal center cells. They frequently occur in patients with Epstein-Barr virus. Interestingly, the age distribution of patients with these lymphomas has two peaks, one between ages 20 and 30 and one greater than 50 years. Patients will have Reed-Sternberg cells, and a contiguous lymph node cells. Patients with Hodgkin's lymphomas will frequently present with painless adenopathy, fever, night sweats, slight weight loss, and pruritus. A physical examination should reveal regional adenopathy and hepatosplenomegaly. The best way to diagnose this condition is to biopsy the largest node, and then perform a chest X-ray. Patients should also consider receiving a bone marrow biopsy and lumbar puncture. As for treatment, localized disease should be given radiation therapy, while more advanced cases require chemotherapy.

Multiple myeloma

Introduction -- Multiple myeloma is a plasma cell disorder, a neoplastic or potentially neoplastic disorder in which there is a proliferation of monoclonal plasma cells of the B-cell series. There are two heavy and two light chains in every immunoglobin. Multiple myeloma is a neoplastic proliferation of plasma cells which leads to a monoclonal light chain or immunoglobin. This condition most frequently affects individuals more than 50 years of age, especially African-Americans and women. Patients with multiple myeloma will typically present with symptoms similar to those of anemia. It is quite common for patients to be frequently infected by encapsulated organisms like Streptococcus pneumoniae.

Symptoms -- Individuals suffering from multiple myeloma are likely to complain of bone pain in their back or ribs, and they may be subject to pathological fractures. It is typical for the symptoms of renal failure and hypercalcemia to be evident. It is also typical for patients to present with neuropathy, spinal cord compression, pallor, fever, bone tenderness, soft tissue masses, bone deformities, and lethargy. A positive diagnosis of multiple myeloma can be made after it is determined that the patient has anemia, proteinuria, elevated erythrocyte sedimentation rate, and a narrow anion gap. Plasma cells will often not appear on a peripheral blood smear. A basic urinalysis may indicate that the patient is suffering from proteinuria.

Diagnosis and treatment -- A diagnosis of multiple myeloma will be supported by serum and urine protein electrophoresis that indicates monoclonal gammopathy, typically IgG, as well as free kappa and lambda light chains, a condition known as Bence Jones proteinuria. Lytic lesions, especially in the axial skeleton, accompanied by osteoporosis and pathological fractures, are often indicated by an X-ray. A bone marrow biopsy will often indicate plasma cells at between 10 and 20 %. As for treatment, patients who present with few symptoms can often be helped by thalidomide. Those patients with acute symptoms, or those patients who for some reason cannot take thalidomide, can receive chemotherapy by means of an alkalyting agent along with prednisone/vincristine, doxorubicin, and dexamethasone. Renal failure can be treated with allopurinol as long as it is not symptomatic; hypercalcemia can be treated with hydration, bisphosphonates, prednisone, and calcitonin.

Anemia

Introduction and symptoms -- Individuals are considered to be anemic when they have a hemoglobin level less than 13.5 g/dL in males and less than 12 g/dL in females. There are a number of different causes of anemia, including red blood cell destruction, diminished red blood cell production, and/or blood loss. Individuals are considered to be at a greater risk of developing anemia when they have a history of bleeding, a record of anemia, or family members who have had anemia. Patients with anemia will typically present with fatigue, dyspnea, and dizziness, and they may have an orthostatic blood pressure. The famous symptom of anemia is an iron deficiency, which may be seen as atrophic glossitis, angular cheleitis, and koilonychias.

Diagnosis -- Anemic individuals will be deficient in vitamin B12, which usually manifests as glossitis and peripheral neuropathy. In order to determine whether a patient is suffering from anemia, it may be necessary to perform a rectal exam with stool guaiac. A diagnosis of anemia is supported when by a complete blood count with indices for red blood cells, including mean corpuscular volume, red cell distribution width, and mean corpuscular hemoglobin concentration. A peripheral blood smear will often indicate the cell types characteristic of anemia: spherocytes indicate G6PD deficiency and membranopathy; blister cells indicate G6PD deficiency; Burr cells indicate acute renal failure and uremia; Heinz bodies indicate thassalemia, hemoglobinopathies, and enzymopathies; schistocytes are characteristic of artificial heart valves and microangiopathic hemolytic anemias; and target cells are characteristic of splenectomy.

Treatment -- The diagnosis of anemia should include a reticulocyte count; the level of reticulocytes will be elevated if the anemia is caused by blood loss or red blood cell destruction, and it will be diminished if it is due to marrow failure. The following studies may be performed to determine the etiology of the anemia: an iron panel; haptoglobin, vitamin B12 and folate levels, bilirubin and lactate dehydrogenase levels; Coombs' test, thyroid-stimulating hormone level, liver function test, and a renal function test. The treatment of anemia depends on the underlying disease. Patients with an iron deficiency should be given supplemental iron; male patients older than 50 should be examined for colorectal cancer. A deficiency in vitamin B12 can be treated with monthly injections, while anemia that is caused by chronic renal disease and anemia caused by chronic disease can be treated with erythropoietin.

MGUS and Waldenstrom's macroglobulinemia

Monoclonal gammopathy of undetermined significance (MGUS) is a plasma cell disorder which is also commonly called benign monoclonal gammopathy. Almost a quarter of those who suffer from this condition will eventually develop myeloma, macroglobulinemia, amyloidosis, or lymphoma. A positive diagnosis of MGUS can be made when the monoclonal protein is evident in the serum without there being any other indication of systemic disease.

Waldenstrom's macroglobulinemia is another plasma disorder, one which commonly affects individuals over the age of forty. A positive diagnosis of this condition can be made after laboratory tests reveal an IgG spike, hyperviscosity, and cold agglutinins.

Glucose-6-phosphate dehydrogenase deficiency: diagnosis

Introduction and symptoms -- Glucose-6-phosphate dehydrogenase deficiency is an x-linked enzyme deficiency that can cause hemolysis that is caused by the release of oxidants from macrophages. G6PD is the most common metabolic of the red blood cell disorders. This kind of acute hemolysis can be caused by infection, diabetic ketoacidosis, and a low pH (also known as acidosis). It can also be the result of certain drugs, like antimalarials, quinolones, sulfa drugs, NSAIDS, nitrofurantoin, fava beans, and excessive vitamin C. Patients suffering from an acute hemolysis will present with jaundice, dark urine, and an acute tubular necrosis a couple of days after exposure. It is also likely that these patients will be suffering from anemia, which is likely to present as pallor, tachycardia, and a systolic ejection murmur.

Diagnosis -- Patients suffering from G6PD deficiency will often present with mesenteric and renal ischemia that result in abdominal and/or back pain. Those patients with chronic hemolysis are also likely to be suffering from heaptosplenomegaly. A positive diagnosis of G6PD deficiency can be made through a G6PD assay, which cannot be made during acute hemolytic episodes or after transfusion. Hemolysis is indicated when a peripheral smear reveals Heinz bodies, microcytosis, and schistocytosis. A complete blood count will typically show anemia and an elevated reticulocyte count. A urinalysis often will indicate hemoglobinuria, elevated levels of urobilinogen, and an acute tubular necrosis. Patients will also often have diminished levels of haptoglobin.

Treatment -- A diagnosis of G6PD deficiency is supported by negative results on the direct and indirect Coombs' tests, as well as by tests that indicate elevated levels of direct and indirect bilirubin. The treatment protocol for patients with G6PD starts with volume loading along with intravenous fluids for renal protection. If it can be done, doctors should remove the oxidative stressor, either by discontinuing the offending drug or treating the infection. If it needs to be done, doctors should conduct red blood cell replacement. Acute crises of G6PD deficiency should resolve themselves after only about a week. This spontaneous resolution is due to new erythrocytes that have increased G6PD activity.

Microangiopathic hemolytic anemia

Microangiopathic hemolytic anemia is a group of disorders in which a coagulopathy is linked with a platelet deficiency and red blood cell hemolysis. This category of conditions includes thrombotic thrombocytopenic purpura, hemolytic-uremic syndrome, and disseminated intravascular coagulation. Thrombotic thrombocytopenic purpura can be identified using the mnemonic FAT RN: fever, anemia, thrombocytopenia, renal dysfunction, and neurological abnormalities. The various conditions grouped under the heading of microangiopathic hemolytic anemia can usually be identified by a peripheral blood smear that indicates schistocytes, or fragmented red blood cells.

Sickle cell disease

Symptoms -- An acute chest syndrome caused by sickle cell disease will manifest as chest pain, pulmonary infiltrate, elevated white blood cell count, and hypoxia. It may be difficult to tell the symptoms of acute chest syndrome from those of pneumonia. An aplastic crisis caused by sickle cell disease is often caused by parvovirus B19 deficiency, while a hemolytic crisis is more commonly associated with G6PD deficiency. During a sequestration crisis, red blood cells will collect in the spleen and can lead to shock and even death. During a splenic crisis, there will be autoinfarction of the spleen, which leads to an elevated risk of osteomyleitis and possible infections by encapsulated organisms.

Introduction -- Sickle cell disease is an autosomal-recessive disease that predominantly affects African-Americans. The carriers of this disease are usually asymptomatic. The signs of sickle cell disease can be remembered with the mnemonic SICKLE: splenomegaly/sludging, infection, cholelithiasis, kidney hematuria, liver congestion/leg ulcers, and eye changes. The disease is typically identified during neonatal screening. The crises of sickle cell disease are usually caused by infection, hypoxia, or dehydration. During an acute crisis, the patient will have arthralgias and pain, which is caused by vascular sludging and thrombosis. This kind of vaso-occlusive crisis can sometimes lead to organ failure, dehydration, fever, and leukocytosis.

Diagnosis and treatment -- A positive diagnosis of sickle cell disease is supported by a blood smear that indicates sickle-shaped cells and Howell-Jolly bodies, which are cytoplasmic leftovers from nuclear chromatin that is usually removed by the spleen. Subsequent blood tests will indicate anemia, an elevated reticulacyte count, and an increased amount of indirect bilirubin. A hemoglobin lectrphoresis will indicate HbS. If the patient is having an acute crisis of sickle cell disease, then he or she should immediately be given fluids and analgesia. The patient should also be given hydroxyurea in order to raise the level of fetal hemoglobin. In order to guard against infection, the patient should be given the influenza and pneumonococcal vaccines, and children under the age of five should be given preventive doses of penicillin. Patients enduring acute chest syndrome need to be given respiratory support and exchange transfusion.

Hemolytic uremic syndrome

Hemolytic uremic syndrome is caused by either a mild viral illness or gastroenteritis accompanied by E. Coli 0157:H7. Patients with this condition will often present with anemia, thrombocytopenia, and acute renal failure. A complete blood count and electrolyte count should reveal anemia and/or thrombocytopenia. The patient will have a normal prothrombin time and partial thromboplastin time, but will have elevated levels of lactate dehydrogenase and a negative result on Coombs' test. A subsequent blood smear will likely indicate schistocytes. The appropriate treatment for hemolytic uremic syndrome is dialysis in order to remedy the acute renal failure.

Disseminated intravascular coagulation

Disseminated intravascular coagulation can be caused by sepsis, a transfusion reaction, neoplasia, trauma, and obstetric complications. The patient will typically present with bleeding at venipuncture sites and epistaxis, as well as digital gangrene and hypotension. A complete blood and electrolyte count will indicate anemia and thrombocytopenia. The patient will have elevated prothrombin time, elevated partial thromboplastin time, and elevated bleeding time. Further lab tests will indicate elevated D-dimer, elevated fibrin split products, and diminished fibrinogen. A blood smear will indicate the presence of schistocytes. The protocol for disseminated intravascular coagulation is to treat the underlying condition, and if necessary to transfuse with platelets and cryopreciptitate.

Thrombotic thrombocytopenic purpura

Thrombotic thrombocytopenic purpura can be caused by HIV infection, pregnancy, or the use of oral contraceptives. Patients with this condition typically present with a pentad of fever, anemia/splenomegaly, thrombocytopenia, acute renal failure, and neurological abnormalities like confusion, headache, and focal problems. A complete blood and electrolyte count will indicate anemia and thrombocytopenia. The patient will typically have normal prothrombin time and partial thromboplastin time, but will have an increased bleeding time. Further test will reveal elevated levels of indirect bilirubin, elevated levels of lactate dehydrogenase, and a negative Coombs' test. It is typical for patients with TTP to have hyaline thrombi in the small vessels without there being any inflammatory changes. A subsequent blood smear will indicate schistocytes. The treatment for TTP includes large-volume plasmapheresis, coriticosteroids, splenectomy, and acetylsalicylic acid.

Beta-thalassemia

Beta-thalassemia occurs as a result of diminished beta-globin chain synthesis. This syndrome is most common in African-Americans, Asians, and individuals from the Mediterranean region. Individuals suffering from beta-thalassemia major, otherwise known as Cooly's anemia, will likely have almost no beta-globin production, and may present with jaundice or splenomegaly. Patients with beta-thalassemia minor will generally present with either very mild or no anemia, and may in fact be asymptomatic carriers. A positive diagnosis of beta-thalassemia is supported when electrophoresis indicates elevated HbF, diminished HbA, and elevated HbA2 measurements. Beta-thalassemia is treated with aggressive transfusions and splenectomy in order to protect existing red blood cells. Some patients may require a bone marrow transplant; they should be given deferoxamine, which increases the urinary excretion of iron in order to prevent complications caused by iron overload. Patients with beta-thalassemia minor should simply avoid oxidative stress.

Alpha-thalassemia

Thalassemia is a cluster of health disorders that are all caused by a diminished amount of synthesis of alpha- and beta-globin protein subunits, of which every human has four and two, respectively. The etiology of alpha-thalassemia is a decreased number of alpha-globin chain syntheses. This condition predominantly affects African-Americans and Asians. The symptoms of alpha-thalassemia are dependent on which of the four foci have been removed or altered. If one of the four has been removed or altered, then the patient may suffer from asymptomatic silent thalassemia; if two, then the patient will carry the thalassemia trait and may suffer from mild anemia; if three, then the patient will have hemoglobin H disease and possibly splenomegaly; and if all four foci have been damaged or removed, then the patient will have hemoglobin Barts, hydrops fetalis, and will probably die soon. A positive diagnosis of alpha-thalassemia can be made after a blood smear indicates that the patient is suffering from microcytic anemia, target cells, hypochromia, and Heinz bodies. Also, if a brilliant cresyl blue stain is taken, then HbH inclusion bodies will be seen. The usual treatment for this condition is periodic blood transfusions.

Polycthemia

Introduction and symptoms -- Polycthemia is a condition in which a person has an elevated red blood cell count and hematocrit levels. This may be a physiological alteration that is made to allow a person to survive in low-oxygen conditions. First-degree polycthemia is idiopathic, but second-degree polycthemia manifests as hypoxemia, meaning that a patient can have chronic obstructive pulmonary disease and lung disease. Individuals with polycthemia will typically present with fever, lethargy, a ruddy complexion, and pruritis. A more thorough physical examination will often reveal vascular sludging, which can often lead to stroke, myocardial infarction, angina, hepatic vein thrombosis, headache, blurred vision, and splenomegaly.

Diagnosis and treatment -- A positive diagnosis of polycthemia is supported by a hematocrit score greater than 50%, increased levels of red blood cell mass, and diminished erythrocyte sedimentation rate. Patients with first-degree polycthemia will have a diminished level of erythropoietin, and patients with second-degree polycthemia will have an elevated level. As for blood counts, both white blood cells and platelets will be elevated, or there may be an elevated level of all blood lines. As for treatment, doctors should consider a serial phlebotomy in order to diminish the blood volume and the risk of vascular events. Doctors should also consider hydroxyurea in order to resolve myelosuppression. It should be noted that the presence of polycthemia vera increases the chances that the patient will convert to chronic myelogenous leukemia, myelofibrosis, or acute myelogenous leukemia.

Transfusion reactions

Blood transfusion is usually performed in order to replace the blood cells or products that an individual has lost because of a severe bleeding episode. An autologous transfusion is a transfusion of one's own blood, and is considered to be the safest method. In cases where a patient suffers from an acute hemolysis during a red blood cell transfusion, he or she may undergo lysis, or destruction of the red blood cells that have been donated. This is most often the result of incompatible blood as a result of errors made by medical staff. The particular type of reaction that is being endured can be diagnosed after the patient's blood type is rechecked against the type of the donor, and disseminated intravascular coagulation labs and cultures of the donor blood are performed.

There are five basic adverse reactions to a blood transfusion. In a hemolytic reaction, the red blood cells are destroyed and hemoglobin is released into the blood plasma. Patients with this kind of reaction will have chest pain, dyspnea, hypotension, and jaundice. Patients suffering from a febrile reaction to donated white blood cells will have a fever, chills, back pain, and a headache. Patients suffering from an allergic reaction to some unknown aspect of the donated blood may manifest urticaria, edema, wheezing, dizziness, and anaplaxia. Patients suffering from hemoglobinuria, in which there is an abnormally high amount of iron absorbed into the blood by the intestinal tract, will manifest acute tubular necrosis, oliguria, and renal failure. If a patient happens to be suffering from an IgG deficiency, then he or she will have an anaphylactic reaction, which may be deadly.

Rejection

A rejection is the body's unwillingness to accept any cells, tissues, or organs that have been transplanted. Rejections may be hyperacute, acute, and chronic.

- A hyperacute rejection happens almost immediately after the introduction of the foreign organic material, and if the patient has preformed antidonor antibodies then the result can be instantaneous vascular thrombi. This can only be solved by removing the new organ.
- An acute rejection will occur between five days and three months after the transplant. This kind of rejection can be diagnosed after a biopsy of the transplanted organ indicates a lymphocyte or antibody-induced reaction with a T-cell graft injury. This can be solved through the introduction of antilymphocyte antibodies, which defuse the body's natural reaction to what it perceives as an invasion.
- A chronic rejection is when the patient gradually loses the use of the transplanted organ months or years after transplantation. This can lead to vascular damage in the form of fibrinoid necrosis, in which the agents that clot the blood are destroyed. Chronic rejections cannot be treated.

Treatment for transfusion reactions

Obviously, the first and most important thing a doctor can do when treating a transfusion reaction is to immediately stop the transfusion. If the patient is having a hemolytic reaction, in which the red blood cells that have been donated are being destroyed, then he or she should be given intravenous fluids and mannitol in order to stave off oliguric renal failure, which is kidney failure in which too little urine is being produced. Patients who are undergoing a severe allergic reaction should be given dipenhydramine or even steroids. A febrile reaction is less severe, and can be guarded against by the administration of acetaminophen. Acetaminophen, known commercially as Tylenol, reduces fever by acting on the portion of the brain that regulates heat.

Bone marrow transplant

In a bone marrow transplant, diseased or damaged bone marrow is replaced with healthy bone marrow. An autologonous bone marrow transplant uses the patient's own bone marrow, while allogeneic bone marrow transplantation uses marrow from an unrelated person. When bone marrow is taken from an identical twin, it is referred to as a syngeneic transplant. One common problem that arises during bone marrow transplantation is called graft vs. host disease, or GVHD. In this scenario, T cells (which are made in the bone marrow) from the donor accumulate in the host and eventually attack the host. Oddly, the T cells that have been transplanted will proliferate to such a great degree that they will consider the host's proteins as foreign.

The adverse condition resulting from bone marrow transplant known as graft versus host disease, or GVHD, can be either acute or chronic. In its acute form, the patient will present with a pruritic maculopopular rash, meaning that the rash will appear as many small and itchy marks on the skin. The patient with acute GVHD may also have liver dysfunction and diarrhea. The chronic form of GVHD is an autoimmune disorder in which the patient may have keratoconjunctivitis sicca, an inflammation of the eye, and lichenoid (small itchy pinkish spots) appearances on the inner lining of the cheeks and lips. The acute form of the disease typically appears within 100 days of the transplantation, and the chronic form appears later than this. The only way to treat this condition is to try and prevent it with cyclosporine, tacrolimus, or methotrexate, a drug that can slow the metabolism of cells.

Neutropenia

Introduction and etiology -- Neutropenia is a significant decrease in the number of neutrophils, or white blood cells. Individuals tend to develop neutropenia when their immune system is generally impaired. The condition is defined clinically as occurring when the level of white blood cells drops below 2000 per cubic millimeter. The patient will begin to develop serious health problems if the level drops below 1000 per cubic millimeter. There are three basic reasons for the development of neutropenia. Either the individual is suffering from marrow failure, has undergone some kind of marrow invasion (as from an infection or cancer), or because normal development has ceased because of a deficiency in folate or vitamin B12.

Diagnosis and treatment -- A patient with neutropenia can have a variety of symptoms, and indeed may be asymptomatic entirely. Some patients will show signs of a serious infection. When marrow failure, marrow invasion, or arrested development are not obvious, then a doctor should perform a bone marrow aspiration, in which a sample of the marrow is removed with a long needle, or a biopsy, in which a tissue sample is removed for examination. The appropriate treatment for neutropenia will depend on the underlying cause. Some patients will require granulocyte colony-stimulating factor, or G-CSF, which boosts the production of tiny sacs that contain micro-organism-destroying enzymes. Other patients may require antibiotics or glucocorticosteroids.

Mental Disorders

Obsessive-compulsive disorder

Obsessive-compulsive personality disorder is a persistent preoccupation with organization and mental/interpersonal control. Obsessions are persistent and involuntary ideas and impulses, and compulsions are repetitive mental or physical acts or behaviors. Four symptoms are required for the diagnosis, including: preoccupation with rules, and details; perfectionism that interferes with progress; excessive devotion to work; counter-productive rigidity about beliefs and morality; inability to throw away old objects; and a reluctance to delegate authority to others. Patients with OCD are typically treated with clomipramine or SSRIs, as well as consistent cognitive-behavioral therapy.

Generalized anxiety disorder

Individuals may be diagnosed with generalized anxiety disorder if they have excessive anxiety about multiple events or activities. This anxiety must have existed for at least six months, and they must be difficult for the individual to control. Also, the anxiety must be disproportionate to the feared event. Anxiety must include at least three of the following: restlessness, difficulty swallowing, feeling on edge, being easily fatigued, difficulty concentrating, irritability, muscle tension, and sleep disturbance. The treatment for generalized anxiety disorder usually ails a multicomponent cognitive-behavioral therapy, often accompanied by the drugs venlafaxine. The SSRI class of antidepressants and the anxiolytic buspirone have both demonstrated success in diminishing the symptoms of GAD. Individuals may develop chronic seizures after long-term use of buspirone.

Panic disorder

Introduction and symptoms -- An individual may have panic disorder if he or she suffers two or more unexpected panic attacks, and one of the attacks is followed by one month of either persistent concern regarding the possibility of another attack or a significant change in behavior related to the attack. Panic disorder is often accompanied by agoraphobia, a fear of places from which escape may be difficult or embarrassing. Panic attacks are brief, defined periods of intense apprehension, fear, or terror. They develop quickly, and usually reach their greatest intensity after about ten minutes. In order for panic disorder to be diagnosed, the attacks must include at least four characteristic symptoms, which include: palpitations or accelerated heart rate, fear of dying, chest pain, nausea, dizziness, derealization, and paresthesia. Although individuals with panic disorder will experience some attacks as a result of traumatic events, at least some of their attacks should be spontaneous.

Diagnosis and treatment -- The most effective treatment for panic attacks and agoraphobia appears to be in vivo exposure with response prevention, otherwise known as flooding. This controlled exposure to the anxiety-inducing situation is typically accompanied by cognitive therapy, relaxation, breathing training, and/or pharmacotherapy. Sometimes benzodiazepines are prescribed in order to provide immediate relief of symptoms, but these drugs are dangerously addictive. Antidepressant medications are often prescribed to relieve the symptoms of panic disorder. If only drug treatment is used, the risk of relapse is very high. Differential diagnoses for panic disorder include social phobia as well as medical conditions like hyperthyroidism, hypoglycemia, cardiac arrhythmia, and mitral valve prolapse. Panic disorder can be distinguished from social phobia by the fact that attacks will sometimes occur while the individual is alone or sleeping.

Specific phobias

Introduction and symptoms -- A specific phobia is a marked and persistent fear of some specific object or situation other than those that are associated with social phobia or agoraphobia. When an individual with a phobia is exposed to the feared object or event, he or she will have a panic attack or some other anxiety response. Adults with a specific phobia should be able to recognize that their fear is irrational and excessive. The onset of a specific phobia is typically in childhood or in the mid-20s. According to the DSM-IV, there are five subtypes of specific phobia: animal, natural environment, situational, blood-injection-injury, and other. The blood-injection-injury subtype has different physical symptoms than the others: individuals with this sort of phobia are likely to have a brief increase in heart rate and blood pressure followed by a drop in both, often ending in the brief loss of consciousness. Other phobic reactions will just entail the increase in heart rate and blood pressure.

Diagnosis and treatment -- There are a number of different treatment protocols for specific phobias, and the method chosen should depend on the preference of the patient as well as the recommendation of the doctor. As with panic disorder, in vivo exposure is considered to be the best treatment for a specific phobia. Some patients will benefit from hypnosis. Relaxation and breathing techniques are also helpful in dispelling fear and controlling physical response. In some cases, low dosages of benzodiazepines, beta-blockers, and the SSRI class of antidepressants may be useful in resolving specific phobias. Medication is not considered to be a permanent solution to phobia, but rather a means of encouraging changes in the patient's pattern of behavior.

Posttraumatic stress disorder

Introduction and symptoms -- An individual has posttraumatic stress disorder (PTSD) if he or she develops characteristic symptoms after exposure to an extreme trauma that entails experiencing or witnessing an event involving death or injury to self or another, or learning about the unexpected or violent death or injury of a family member or friend. This event must elicit a reaction of intense fear, helplessness, or horror in order for the diagnosis to be made. The characteristic symptoms of PTSD are: persistent reexperiencing of the event; persistent avoidance of stimuli associated with the trauma; and persistent symptoms of increased arousal (for example difficulty concentrating, staying awake, or falling asleep). These symptoms must have been present for at least a month; symptoms may not begin until three or more months after the event.

Treatment -- At present, the preferred treatment for PTSD is a comprehensive cognitive-behavioral approach that includes exposure, cognitive restructuring, and anxiety management, among other techniques. Some studies suggest that SSRIs can be helpful in treating some of the symptoms of PTSD as well as many of the comorbid conditions. As for other medication, many of those diagnosed with PTSD are prescribed beta-blockers, benzodiazepines, and alpha2-agonists. A controversial therapy used to treat PTSD is eye movement desensitization and reprocessing; the positive benefits of this therapy may be more to do with the exposure that goes along with it than with the eye movements themselves.

Social phobia

The characteristics of social phobia are a marked and persistent fear of social situations or situation in which the individual may be called upon to perform. Typically, the individual will fear the criticism and evaluation of others. The response to the feared situation is an immediate panic attack. Individuals with social phobia will either avoid the feared situation or will endure it with much distress. Adults should be able to recognize that their fear is excessive and irrational. As with other phobias, social phobia is best treated with exposure in combination with social skills and cognitive therapy. The medication that is most often prescribed in order to treat social phobias are SSRI antidepressants, benzodiazepines, and in particular beta-blockers, which seem to be especially good at diminishing performance anxiety.

Dementia

Introduction and symptoms -- Dementia is any impairment in cognitive functioning that is acquired by the individual. Individuals who suffer from dementia will manifest a few cognitive deficits, most notably memory impairment, aphasia, apraxia, agnosia, and/or impaired executive functioning. Depending on the etiology of the dementia, these deficits may get progressively worse or may be permanent. Demented individuals often have both anterograde and retrograde amnesia, meaning that they find it difficult both to learn new information and to recall previously learned information. There may be a decrease in language skill, specifically manifested in an inability to recall the names of people or things. Individuals may also have a hard time performing routine motor programs, and may be unable to recognize familiar people and places. Abstract thinking, planning, and initiating complex behaviors are difficult for demented individuals.

Diagnosis and treatment -- Dementia can be diagnosed after close examination of the patient and careful consideration of history. The treatable causes of dementia, like infection and exogenous causes can be excluded by the performance of a complete blood count, rapid plasma reagin, thyroid function test, and HIV test. Dementia differs from delirium in that the patient is usually alert and undergoing a gradual dimunition in cognitive function. Also, a demented individual will rarely hallucinate. The treatment of dementia involves tailoring the patient's environment to his or her dysfunction by making it highly structured and user-friendly. Agitated patients can be given antipsychotics, though benzodiazepines should be avoided.

Delirium: introduction, symptoms

Introduction and symptoms -- Delirium is an ephemeral interruption of normal consciousness. Delirium, like dementia, is characterized by a clinically significant deficit in cognition or memory as compared to previous functioning. In order for delirium to be diagnosed, the individual must have disturbances in consciousness and either a change in personality or the development of perceptual abnormalities. These changes in cognition may appear as losses of memory, disorientation in space and time, and impaired language. The perceptual abnormalities associated with delirium include hallucinations and illusions. Delirium usually develops over a few hours or days, and may vary in intensity over the course of the days and weeks. If the cause of the delirium is alleviated, it may disappear for an extended period of time.

Diagnosis and treatment -- There are five groups of people who are at a high risk of delirium: elderly people; those who have a diminished cerebral reserve due to dementia, stroke, or some other medical condition; post-cardiotomy patients; burn patients; and people who are withdrawing from a drug dependency. The diagnosis of delirium can be made after pulse oximetry, vital signs, and glucose levels have been checked. A history of the patient's recent illness and medication should be taken. Delirium is differentiated from dementia in that it can often be reversed. The treatment for delirium usually aims at curing the underlying cause of the disorder and reducing the agitated behavior. Antipsychotic drugs can be good for reducing agitation, delusions, and hallucinations, while providing a clam environment can decrease the appearance of agitation.

Major depressive disorder

Symptoms -- The two major symptoms of major depressive disorder are a depressed mood and/or a loss of interest in activities that formerly brought pleasure. This condition must persist for at least two weeks for the event to be classified as a major depressive episode. Individuals suffering from major depressive disorder often also suffer from chronic illness and increased stress. At least five of the following symptoms will be present: depressed mood most of the time; diminished interest or pleasure in all activities; feelings of worthlessness or inappropriate guilt; psychomotor agitation or retardation; loss or increase in appetite and significant weight loss or gain; fatigue or loss of energy; insomnia or hypersomnia; reduced ability to concentrate; and suicidal ideation.

Treatment -- The typical treatment program for major depressive disorder combines antidepressant drugs and psychotherapy. There are three classes of antidepressant medication that are commonly prescribed. Selective serotonin reuptake inhibitors (SSRIs) are prescribed for melancholic depressives; they have a lower incidence of serious adverse side effects than do tricyclics. Tricylclics (TCAs), however, are the most commonly prescribed drug for classic depression: that is, depression involving vegetative bodily symptoms, a worsening of symptoms in the morning, and the acute onset and short duration of moderate symptoms. Finally, monamine oxidase inhibitors are prescribed as a last resort for patients who have an unorthodox depression that includes phobias, panic attacks, increased appetite, hypersomnia, and a mood that worsens as the day goes on. Electroconvulsive therapy has had good results treating endogenous forms of depression that include delusions or suicidal ideation. Some patients have suffered temporary retrograde and anterograde amnesia after ECT, but this problem can be mitigated by limiting the ECT to the right, nondominant hemisphere.

Bipolar disorders

Introduction and symptoms -- Bipolar I disorders include the occurrence of one or more manic or mixed episodes, with or without a history of one or more major depressive episodes. There are a few subtypes of Bipolar I disorder: single manic episode, most recent episode manic, most recent episode hypomanic, most recent episode mixed, and most recent episode depressed. Bipolar II disorder, on the other hand, can be diagnosed when a person has had at least one major depressive episode and one hypomanic episode. Bipolar II disorder is distinguished by the fact that the individual has never had either a manic or a mixed episode. The presentation of the manic state common to bipolar disorder includes distractibility, sexual indiscretion, talkativeness, grandiosity, and insomnia. Males and females develop Bipolar I disorder equally, but Bipolar II is much more common for females. On average, the age of onset for the first manic episode is the early 20s.

Diagnosis and treatment -- Bipolar disorder can be diagnosed when the patient has one or more manic episodes a week, and has a persistently elevated or irritable mood. The most effective treatment for Bipolar I and II is lithium. This drug seems to reduce manic symptoms and eliminate mood swings for over half of the people that take it. One major problem with lithium is that it works so well that many patients will consider themselves cured and stop taking it, causing a relapse. Pharmacotherapy is most effective when combined with psychotherapy. Some patients do not respond to lithium treatment, and are given anti-seizure drugs like carbamazepine or divalproex sodium. These drugs are also often used in lieu of lithium for patients who have rapid cycling or dysphoric mania.

Paranoid personality disorder

Paranoid personality disorder is a pervasive pattern of distrust and suspiciousness that involves believing the actions and thoughts of other people to be directed antagonistically against oneself. In order to make the diagnosis, the individual must have at least four of the following symptoms: suspects that others are somehow harming him or her; doubts the trustworthiness of others; reluctant to confide in others; suspicious without justification about the fidelity of one's partner. One of the main problems in the treatment of paranoid personality disorder is that the patient will probably distrust doctors and therefore will be unlikely to pursue medical attention on his or her own.

Schizotypal personality disorder

Schizotypal personality disorder is pervasive social deficits and oddities of cognition, perception, and behavior. A diagnosis requires four of the following: ideas of reference; odd beliefs; magical thinking; bodily illusions; suspiciousness; social anxiety; inappropriate or constricted affect; and peculiarities in behavior or appearance. Magical thinking is when an individual attributes effects to impossible causes, and/or believes their own actions to have supernatural effects. In order to treat a schizotypal patient, a doctor should maintain as professional a tone as possible, and should avoid making light of the patient's irregular thinking. Clarity and accuracy are the most important qualities of effective treatment.

Schizoid personality disorder

Schizoid personality disorder is a pervasive lack of interest in relationships with others, as well as a limited range of emotional expression in contacts with others. A schizoid type is colloquially known as a loner. For a diagnosis, at least four symptoms must be present, including: avoidance of or displeasure in close relationships; always chooses solitude; little interest in sexual relationships; takes pleasure in few activities; indifference to praise or criticism; and emotional coldness or detachment. Schizoid patients are likely to be suspicious of medical practitioners, so the appropriate strategy for a doctor is to remain clear and honest without trying to attain too great of an intimacy with the patient.

Borderline personality disorder

Borderline personality disorder is a pervasive pattern of instability in social relationships, self-image, and affect, coupled with marked impulsivity. A diagnosis requires five symptoms, which include: frantic efforts to avoid being abandoned; a pattern of unstable and intense personal relationships, in which there is alternation between idealization and devaluation; instability in self-image; potentially self-destructive impulsivity in at least two areas; recurrent suicide threats or gestures; affective instability; and chronic feelings of emptiness. Patients with borderline personality disorder may attempt to manipulate their treatment, and should be treated with consistency and firmness.

Antisocial personality disorder

Antisocial personality disorder is a Cluster B personality disorder, meaning that it has to do with dramatic, emotional, or erratic behaviors. It is a general lack of concern for the rights and feelings of others. In order to receive this diagnosis, the individual must be at least 18, have had a history of conduct disorder before age 15, and must have shown at least three of the following symptoms before the age of 15: failure to conform to social laws and norms; deceitfulness; impulsivity; reckless disregard for the safety of self and others; consistent irresponsibility; and a lack of remorse. This disorder may also include an inflated opinion of self, superficial charm, and a lack of empathy for others. Patients with antisocial personality disorder should be approached with consistency and fairness above all else.

Narcissistic personality disorder

Narcissistic personality disorder is grandiose behavior along with a lack of empathy and a need for admiration. The individual must exhibit five symptoms for diagnosis, including:

grandiose sense of self-importance; fantasies of own power and beauty; belief in personal uniqueness; need for excessive admiration; sense of entitlement; exploitive of others; and a lack of empathy. Narcissistic personality disorder is one of the cluster B personality disorders, a group distinguished by wild and unpredictable behavior. Narcissistic patients may attempt to influence their care providers, so treatment should include firm and consistent rules. The ego of a narcissist is very sensitive, so therapy should avoid direct challenges.

Histrionic personality disorder

Histrionic personality disorder is excessive emotionality and attention-seeking behavior. Five symptoms like the following must be present for a diagnosis: annoyance or discomfort when not receiving attention; inappropriate sexual provocation; rapidly shifting and shallow emotions; vague and impressionistic speech; exaggerated expression of emotion; easily influenced by others; and misapprehension of relationships as more intimate than they are. Histrionic personality disorder is considered to be one of the Cluster B personality disorders, meaning that behavior may be wild and unpredictable. Patients should be treated fairly, but should not be allowed to manipulate the terms of their treatment. Consistency is important when treating individuals with histrionic personality disorder.

Dependent personality disorder

Dependent personality disorder is an excessive need to be taken care of. The diagnosis requires five symptoms from among: difficulty making decision without advice; need for others to assume responsibility for one's actions; fear of disagreeing with others; difficulty self-initiating projects; and feelings of helplessness or discomfort when alone. Effort should be made to separate abnormal behavior in this vein from behavior that is culturally acceptable to the individual. Patients with a dependent personality disorder may attempt to sabotage their own treatment, or may indicate assent to treatment without actually committing. In order to avoid alienating a patient with this condition, doctors should seek to establish a collaborative relationship.

Avoidant personality disorder

Avoidant personality disorder is a cluster C personality, meaning that it involves the feelings of anxiety or fearfulness. It is a pervasive pattern of social inhibition, feelings of inadequacy, and hypersensitivity to negative evaluation. A person with this diagnosis will exhibit at least four symptoms like: avoiding work or school activities that involve interpersonal contact; being unwilling to associate with any person who is not sure to approve of them; preoccupation with concerns about being criticized or rejected; conception of self as socially inept, inferior, or unappealing to others; and a general reluctance to take personal risks or engage in dangerous behavior. Patients with this disorder should be given strong recommendations, but should not be forced to do anything.

Schizophrenia

Introduction -- Schizophrenia is the umbrella term for a variety of brain diseases that are marked by alterations in personality, agitation, catatonia, psychosis, and social withdrawal. Males and females are just as likely to develop this disorder, which affects about 1% of the population. Males will typically develop schizophrenia earlier than females. This is a very serious condition, as almost one in ten schizophrenics will commit suicide. It is not entirely known what causes schizophrenia, although current speculation focuses on abnormalities in neurotransmission and in more general abnormalities in brain physiology like frontal hypoactivity and limbic hyperactivity.

Symptoms -- The symptoms of schizophrenia may be positive, negative, or disorganized. The positive symptoms are delusions and hallucinations. Delusions are false beliefs that are held despite clear evidence to the contrary. The delusions suffered by a schizophrenic usually fall into one of three categories: persecutory, in which the person believes that someone or thing is out to get him or her; referential, in which the person believes that messages in the public domain (as for instance song lyrics or newspaper articles) are specifically directed at him or her; and bizarre, in which the person imagines that something impossible has happened. The most common sensory mode for hallucinations is sound, specifically the audition of voices.

For many psychologists, the tell-tale characteristic of schizophrenia is disorganized speech. Disorganized speech may be manifested as incoherence, free associations that make little sense, and random responses to direct questions. Disorganized behavior is manifested as a shabby or unkempt appearance; inappropriate sexual behavior; unpredictable agitation; or catatonia and decreased motor activity. The negative symptoms of schizophrenia are restrictions in the range of emotions; reduced body language; lack of a facial expression; lack of coherent thoughts; inability to make conversation; and avolition (the inability to set goals or to work in a rational, programmatic manner).

Diagnosis -- In order to be diagnosed with schizophrenia, an individual must have a continuous disturbance of more than six months that includes one or more of the following active-phase symptoms: delusions; hallucinations; disorganized sleep; severely disorganized or catatonic behavior; and negative symptoms. Also, the afflicted individual must be suffering impairment in his or her performance at home, work, interpersonal life, or self-care. Schizophrenia is considered to be a psychotic disorder. Psychotic disorders are those that feature one or more of the following: delusions; hallucinations; disorganized speech or thought; and disorganized or catatonic behavior.

Treatment -- Treatment for schizophrenia begins with the administration of antipsychotic medication. These drugs are very effective at diminishing the positive symptoms of schizophrenia, though their results vary from person to person. Antipsychotics may have strong side effects, however, including tardive dyskinesia. Medication is more effective when it is taken in combination with psychosocial intervention. Many schizophrenics are prone to relapse if they receive a great deal of criticism from family members, so it may be a good idea to initiate family therapy in which the level of expressed emotion in the family is discussed. Recovering schizophrenics also benefit from social skills training and help with employment.

ADHD

Introduction -- Attention-deficit hyperactivity disorder is a pattern of inattention combined with hyperactivity or impulsivity. There are slightly higher rates of the disorder among biological relatives than among the general population, and there are higher rates among identical than fraternal twins. ADHD has also been associated with some structural abnormalities in the brain, like subnormal activity in the frontal cortex and basal ganglia, and a relatively small caudate nucleus, globus pallidus, and prefrontal cortex. The symptoms of ADHD are likely to vary widely depending on the individual's environment. Repetitive or boring environments seem to encourage symptoms, as do those in which the individual is given no chance to interact.

Symptoms and diagnosis -- Attention-deficit/hyperactivity disorder, commonly known as ADHD, can be diagnosed only if an individual displays at least six symptoms of inattention or hyperactivity-impulsivity. The symptoms of inattention include difficulty sustaining tasks or play activities; not listening when addressed directly; failing to finish schoolwork or chores; being easily distracted by extraneous stimuli; and forgetfulness. The symptoms of hyperactivity-impulsivity include frequent fidgeting or squirming in a seat; running or climbing in inappropriate situations; difficulty in playing quietly; excessive talking; interrupting; and intruding on others. In order for ADHD to be diagnosed, these symptoms must have had an onset before the age of 7, and must have persisted for at least 6 months.

Treatment -- Somewhat counterintuitively, central nervous system stimulants like methylphenidate (Ritalin) have had success in treating the symptoms of ADHD. Research has consistently shown that pharmacotherapy works best when it is combined with psychosocial intervention. Many teachers have used the basic elements of classroom management to control the symptoms of ADHD. This involves laying out clear guidelines and contingencies for behavior, so that students do not have to speculate on what will happen in class or what they should be doing. Therapy that tries to increase the child's ability to self-regulate behavior has been shown to be less successful. It is always helpful when parents are involved in the treatment program.

Autism

Introduction -- Autism is known as a pervasive developmental disorder because it entails a severe and pervasive impairment in communication and social interaction. Autism is frequently suspected first when an infant does not respond to his or her caregiver in the age-appropriate manner. Autistic babies will not be interested in cuddling, will not smile, and will not respond to a familiar voice. This last symptom often causes autistic babies to be misdiagnosed with hearing problems as infants.

Symptoms -- In order to diagnose autism, there must be at least six classic symptoms from three categories, with at least two symptoms from the first category and one from each of the second two categories. These symptoms must have had an onset before the age of three.

- The first category is qualitative impairment in social interaction, which includes the absence of developmentally appropriate peer relationships; a lack of social or emotional reciprocity; and a marked impairment in nonverbal behavior.
- The second category of autism symptoms, of which an individual must display at least one to be diagnosed with autism, is qualitative impairment in communication. This includes a delay or lack of development in spoken language; marked impairment in the ability to initiate or sustain conversation; stereotyped or repetitive use of language or idiosyncratic language; and a lack of developmentally appropriate play.
- The third category of symptoms is restricted, repetitive, and stereotyped behavior, interests, and activities. These include a preoccupation with one or more stereotyped and restricted patterns of interest; inflexible adherence to nonfunctional routines or rituals; stereotyped and repetitive motor mannerisms; and a persistent preoccupation with the parts of objects. There are some very noticeable, specific behavior patterns that are characteristic of autism. Individuals with autism make little eye contact and generally seem uninterested in the presence of others. As infants, they will rarely reach out to a caregiver. One common feature of autistic speech is echolalia, the imitation and repetition of the words of others. Oftentimes, autistic individuals will become obsessively interested in a very narrow subject, like astronomy or basketball. They are likely to place a heavy emphasis on routine and consistency, and may react violently to changes in their normal environment. There are a few motions typical of autism: hand-flapping, rocking, and spinning are among them. The majority of individuals with autism have an IQ in the mentally retarded range.

Treatment -- As for treatment, the most successful psychotherapeutic interventions are those which focus on teaching autistic individuals the practical skills they will need to survive independently. Therapy should also include development of social skills and the reduction of undesirable behavior. Autistic individuals who reach a moderate level of functioning can be given direct vocational training. Unfortunately, even a small degree of improvement in autism takes a great deal of work. Only one-third of autistic children will achieve some independence as adults. The best chance for future independence is in those autistic individuals who have developed the ability to communicate verbally by age 5 or 6, and have an IQ over 70.

Conduct Disorder

Treatment -- There are a number of different opinions on how to treat Conduct Disorder. Research suggests that interventions are most successful when they are administered to preadolescents and include the immediate family members. Some therapists have developed programs of parent therapy to help adults manage the antisocial behavior of their children, as this has been demonstrated to have good success. Most programs advise rewarding good behavior and consistently punishing bad behavior. It is important that Conduct Disorder be treated as quickly as possible, so that it does not become antisocial personality disorder later in life. Part of the treatment for this problem may include understanding and removing the source of stress for the patient.

Diagnosis -- Individuals with Conduct Disorder persistently violate either the rights of others or age-appropriate rules. They will also tend to have little remorse about their behavior, and in ambiguous situations they will be likely to interpret the behavior of other people as hostile or threatening. Conduct Disorder is more likely to occur in males, especially those with a history of abuse. Individuals are diagnosed as having Conduct Disorder when they display three symptoms over the course of a year. The symptoms of Conduct Disorder fall into four main categories: aggression to people or animals; destruction of property; deceitfulness or theft; and serious violations of rules. Childhood-onset Type is a subset of Conduct Disorder in which the onset of symptoms is before age 10; if the onset is after age 10, the subset is Adolescent-onset Type.

Mental retardation

Introduction -- Mental retardation is the result of a chromosomal abnormality, and is more likely to affect impoverished males. The first signs of mental retardation are a lack of interest in environmental stimuli and impaired motor development. Normally, an infant will make eye contact while nursing, and will respond to voices or movements; retarded children may not do either of these. Contrary to the general opinion, mild mental retardation is not necessarily a permanent condition. After much effort and treatment, an individual may no longer meet the diagnostic criteria for mental retardation. Very few (approximately 5%) of all cases of mental retardation are hereditary. The differential diagnosis for mental retardation may be Borderline Intellectual Functioning if the individual has an IQ between 70 and 85. Individuals with an IQ in this range who also have severe adaptive disabilities will be better classified as mentally retarded.

Diagnosis and treatment -- Mental retardation is usually diagnosed during infancy, childhood, or adolescence. In order to be diagnosed with mental retardation, an individual must meet three criteria. First, he or she must function intellectually at a level that is way below average. An IQ of 70 or lower is considered to be consistent with mental retardation. Second, the individual must have concurrent deficits or impairments in at least two other areas, for instance social skills, self-direction, or work. Finally, the onset of the condition must have occurred before the age of 18. Individual with mental retardation may be either mildly retarded (IQ 50-70); moderately retarded (IQ 35-55); severely retarded (IQ 20-40); or profoundly retarded (IQ less than 25). The only treatment for mental retardation is family counseling and speech, physical, and vocational therapy.

Tourette's Disorder

Introduction and symptoms -- Tourette's Disorder is characterized by the presence of at least one vocal tic and multiple motor tics that appear simultaneously or at different times and appear before the age of 18. Tics are defined in the DSM as "sudden, rapid, recurrent, nonrhythmic, stereotyped motor movements or vocalizations that feel irresistible yet can be suppressed for varying lengths of time." Individuals with Tourette's Disorder are also likely to have obsessions and compulsions, as well as high levels of hyperactivity, impulsivity, and distractibility. Some of the other tics that are common to all tic disorders (like chronic motor or vocal tic disorder, or transient tic disorder) are blinking, grimacing, echokinesis (imitating the movements of another person), grunting, barking, echolalia, coprolalia (repeating obscene words), and palilalia (repeating one's own words).

Diagnosis and treatment -- Most successful treatments for Tourette's Disorder include pharmacotherapy. In particular, the antipsychotics haloperidol and pimozide have been successful in relieving the symptoms of this disorder. These drugs inhibit the flow of dopamine in the brain; their success has led many scientists to speculate that Tourette's Disorder is caused by an excess of dopamine. In some cases, psychostimulant drugs amplify the tics displayed by the individual. In these cases, a doctor may treat the hyperactivity and inattention of Tourette's with clonidine or desipramine. The former of these is a drug usually used to treat hypertension, while the latter is typically used as an antidepressant.

Substance-induced disorders

In order for a substance-induced disorder to be diagnosed, there must be clear evidence that the symptoms are related to substance use. There are a number of different ways this can be ascertained: direct physical evidence; evaluation of the relation in time between substance use and the onset of symptoms; the cessation of symptoms after a period of abstinence; the presence of symptoms that are not associated with any other mental disorder; and/or direct empirical evidence of a relationship between the substance and the observed symptoms. Individuals may have substance-induced disorders related to the abuse of alcohol, amphetamines, cocaine, and caffeine, among other substances.

Substance abuse

Substance abuse is characterized by a set of maladaptive behaviors associated with substance use. In order to be diagnosed with substance abuse, an individual must display at least one of the following symptoms during a year-long period: recurrent substance use that results in a failure to fulfill major role obligations at home, school, or work; repeated use of a substance in situations in which use is known to be physically hazardous; recurrent substance-related legal problems; and continued use despite having persistent or recurrent social or interpersonal problems that are caused or exacerbated by the substance. Any of these problems can lead to a diagnosis of substance abuse.

Amphetamine or cocaine -- The characteristics of amphetamine and cocaine intoxication are maladaptive behavioral and psychological changes, including euphoria, hyperactivity, grandiosity, confusion, anger, paranoid ideation, and auditory hallucinations; tachycardia; elevated or lowered blood pressure; dilated pupils; perspiration or chills; nausea or vomiting; weight loss; psychomotor agitation; muscular weakness; confusion; and seizures. The symptoms of amphetamine and cocaine withdrawal are dysphoric mood; fatigue; vivid and unpleasant dreams; insomnia or hypersomnia; increased appetite; psychomotor agitation or retardation. After a period of prolonged or heavy use, the individual may experience a period of intense depression.

Alcoholism -- Alcoholism is more common in males than females, especially between the ages of 20 and 35. The symptoms of alcohol intoxication include: maladaptive behavior and psychological changes; slurred speech; poor coordination; unsteady gait; nystagmus; impaired attention and memory; stupor or coma. The symptoms associated with alcohol withdrawal are: autonomic hyperactivity (including sweating and tachycardia); hand tremors; insomnia; nausea and vomiting; transient illusions or hallucinations; anxiety; psychomotor agitation; and, after periods of prolonged or heavy use, grand mal seizures. Diagnosed alcoholics should be given multivitamins, folic acid, and a benzodiazepine taper in order to battle the symptoms of withdrawal.

Anorexia nervosa

Introduction and symptoms -- The demographic at most risk of anorexia nervosa is wealthy females with low self-esteem. The characteristics of anorexia nervosa are: the refusal to maintain a healthy weight; a fear of gaining weight; significant disturbance in the perception of one's own weight; and, among females, amenorrhea. A general standard used to determine the minimum healthy body weight is that it should be at least 85% of the norm for the individual's height and weight. Restricting type anorexics lose weight through fasting, dieting, and excessive exercise. Binging/purging types do so by eating a great deal and then either vomiting it or inducing immediate defecation with laxatives. Anorexics may remain preoccupied with food. The physical symptoms of starvation are constipation, cold intolerance, lethargy, and bradycardia. The physical problems associated with purging are anemia, impaired renal function, cardiac abnormalities, dental problems, and osteoporosis.

Treatment -- It is essential that anyone suspected of suffering from anorexia nervosa receive immediate treatment, as more than one in ten of those who have this disorder will commit suicide or die from medical complications. The immediate goal of any treatment program for anorexia nervosa is to help the patient gain weight. Sometimes this requires hospitalization in order to stabilize the patient's weight. Cognitive therapy is also often employed to correct the individual's misconceptions about healthy weight and nutrition. Some of the dangerous complications of anorexia nervosa include mitral valve prolapse, hypotension, arrhythmia, nephrolithiasis, osteoporosis, pancytopenia, thyroid abnormalities, and multiple stress fractures.

Bulimia nervosa

Introduction and symptoms -- As with anorexia, the vast majority of bulimics are female. The onset is typically in late adolescence or early adulthood, and may follow a period of dieting. There are indications of a genetic etiology for bulimia. Also, there are links between bulimia and low levels of the endogenous opioid beta-endorphin, as well as low levels of serotonin and norepinephrine. The characteristics of bulimia nervosa are: recurrent episodes of binge eating in which the individual feels out of control; unhealthy behavior aimed at compensating for these binges (as for instance, vomiting); and a harsh conception of self that is largely based on weight. These binges are often caused by interpersonal stress and may entail a staggering caloric intake.

Diagnosis and treatment -- Binge eating and compensatory behavior must have occurred at least twice a month for three months in order for the diagnosis to be made. The main point of any treatment for bulimia is encouraging the individual to get control of eating, and modifying unhealthy beliefs about body shape and nutrition. Treatment often involves cognitive-behavioral techniques like self-monitoring, stimulus control, cognitive restructuring, problem-solving, and self-distraction. Some antidepressants, like imipramine, have been effective at reducing instances of binging and purging. The medical complications associated with bulimia are fluid and electrolyte disturbances, metabolic alkalosis, metabolic acidosis, dental problems, and menstrual abnormalities

Nervous System Diseases

Cerebral stroke

Introduction and symptoms -- A stroke can be either a sudden or a gradual onset of neurological symptoms that are caused by a disruption in the supply of blood to the brain. There are three major causes of stroke. An embolism is the sudden blockage of an artery by material from somewhere else in the blood stream. A thrombosis is a blockage of an artery by a blood clot. Third cause of stroke is hemorrhage. High blood pressure and atherosclerosis are the two most common risk factors for stroke, although people are also more subject to strokes when they smoke or have diabetes. The general symptoms of stroke are contralateral hemiplegia, hemianaesthesia of the face, arms, and legs, and contralateral visual field loss.

Diagnosis and treatment -- In order to diagnose and assess the severity of a cerebral stroke, a doctor needs to perform a CT scan without contrast as well as an MRI. If the patient is suspected of having extracranial disease, then a MRA or carotid ultrasound should be performed; if the patient is suspected of having intercranial disease, then a MRA or transcranial Doppler should be performed. As for treatment, patients who have suffered acute strokes need to be monitored to ensure that their brain does not swell and that they do not develop any hernias. It is essential that hypotension and hypoxemia be avoided during treatment. The patient's systolic blood pressure should be maintained about 20 mmHg higher than normal.

Subdural hematoma

A subdural hematoma occurs between the brain and its covering, which is the dura. It most often occurs after head trauma, such as the rupture of bridging veins, which happen often in the elderly and alcoholics. In infants, a subdural hematoma can induce the fontanel to bulge, which increases the head circumference. Symptoms include headache, slurred speech, impaired gait, contralateral hemiparesis, and may appear as dementia in the elderly. To diagnose, a CT will demonstrate a crescent-shaped, concave hyperdensity that does not cross the midline. If this is a chronic condition, the subdural blood may regress on its own, otherwise, trepanation will drain the excess blood. This condition can progress to coma and even lead to death.

Subarachnoid hemorrhage (SAH)

Usually the result of an artery breaking open into the brain, a subarachnoid hemorrhage can be caused by trauma, a ruptured aneurysm, AVM, or trauma to the circle of Willis. The resulting blood flows into the subarachnoid, which is the space between the arachnoid and the pia matter (the innermost membrane around the central nervous system). Patients may present with an acute-onset, extremely painful headache, as well as neck stiffness, fever, nausea or vomiting, and altering degrees of consciousness. To diagnose, perform a head CT without contrast to look for blood in the subarachnoid space, and an LP if the CT is negative, looking for RBCs, xanthochromia, and increased ICP. Perform a four-vessel angiography once

SAH is diagnosed. SAH requires a neurosurgical procedure. To treat, prevent rebleeding, prevent vasospasm and seizures, and lower ICP.

Parenchymal hemorrhage

Some risk factors that lead to a parenchymal hemorrhage include hypertension, tumor, vascular malformations, and amyloid angiopathy (for the elderly). Patient may present with lethargy and headache, focal motor and sensory deficits, and obtundation (mental dullness, sometimes caused by head trauma) is possible. To diagnose, perform a noncontrast head CT to look for mass effect or edema that could predict herniation, the abnormal protrusion of tissue through an opening. In order to treat this type of hemorrhage, elevate the head of the bed and prevent seizures. A parenchymal hemorrhage may require surgery if there is a mass effect. There are several types of herniation that can happen, among them central, uncal, sufalcine, and tonsillar.

Epidural hematoma

An epidural hematoma occurs between the skull and the dura. It is usually caused by a lateral skull fracture (the result of a blow to the head), which leads to a tear of the middle meningeal artery. The patient will experience a change in mental status in anywhere from minutes to hours, with a lucid interval, as opposed to the days to weeks for which a patient with subdural hematoma will undergo a changed mental status. Then the patient will experience headache, progressive obtundation, hemiparesis, ending with a "blown pupil," which is fixed and dilated. Using a CT scan to diagnose, the physician will see a lens-shaped, convex hyperdensity limited by the sutures. The treatment for this condition is trepanation, to be performed in neurosurgery.

Headaches

Cluster, tension and sinus -- A cluster headache is characterized by excruciating, burning pain that occurs in clusters over a 2-3 month period. The pain is often centered behind one of the eyes, though it may spread to the face and/or temple. Acute cluster headaches may be treated with oxygen, ergots, or corticosteroids. Tension headaches are characterized by nonthrobbing pain on both sides of the head, at the back of the neck, and/or in the face. A tension headache may feel like a band of pressure around the head, almost like a tight hat. Although the traditional view was that tension headaches were caused by stress and muscle tension, it is now believed that they may also be caused by the dilation of blood vessels in the skull. The final kind of non-migraine headache is the sinus headache, which feels like pressure in the sinus cavity. This kind of headache may be caused by infection of the frontal sinuses.

Migraines -- Migraine headaches are severe, recurrent headaches that are usually restricted to one side of the head. Migraine headaches throb with pain, and are frequently accompanied by nausea, vomiting, diarrhea or constipation, and extreme sensitivity to light, noise, and odors. Any motion tends to make the headache much worse. A classic migraine begins with an aura, or focal onset, which alerts the individual that a migraine is about to occur. A common migraine does not have an aura, but may be preceded by gastrointestinal difficulties. There is considerable debate about the etiology of migraines, but most research suggests that they arise out of problems with the constriction and dilation of blood vessels in the brain. Anti-inflammatory drugs and SSRIs have been useful in treating migraines, as have beta-blockers.

Seizures

Tonic-clonic seizures -- Tonic-clonic seizures, also known as grand mal seizures, are the most outwardly apparent form of seizure. They are known as tonic-clonic seizures because they feature a period of immobility followed by a period of uncontrolled jerking. Some individuals will report having felt an aura before the onset of a tonic-clonic seizure. These seizures often feature incontinence and tongue-biting, and may last a few seconds or several minutes. These seizures can be treated with phenytoin, fosphenytoin, or valproate. If the patient has a series of these seizures, or if a single seizure does not resolve, the patient should be hospitalized immediately. These seizures should be distinguished from absence (petit mal) seizures, in which the individual has minor episodes of impaired consciousness that may pass unnoticed. These are typically treated with ethosuxamide.

Partial seizures -- Partial seizures originate in a specific region in one of the cerebral hemispheres and should not result in a loss of consciousness. A simple partial seizure entails jerky limb movements while normal consciousness is maintained. A complex partial seizure features a slightly impaired level of consciousness and the presence of visual or auditory hallucinations. In order to make a positive diagnosis of partial seizure, a doctor should obtain an electroencephalogram, complete blood count, erythrocyte sedimentation rate, and liver function test. The treatment for partial seizures usually focuses on identifying and treating the underlying causes; patients who have a series of these seizures may be given carbamazepine, phenobarbitol, and valproic acid.

Myasthenia Gravis

Myasthenia gravis is an autoimmune neuromuscular disorder that results from antibodies binding to postsynaptic acetylcholine (ACh) receptors. This typically strikes young adult women and is associated with thyrotoxicosis, thymoma, and other autoimmune disorders. Patient may present with fatigable ptosis or double vision, fatigue, and muscle exhaustion. These symptoms often worsen over the course of the day. A myasthenic crisis is a respiratory compromise or aspiration, both of which are rare but can be deadly. To diagnose, the edrophonium, or Tensilon test, uses anticholinesterase to provide amelioration of the symptoms. A similar diagnostic tool uses an ice pack to cover an eye for five minutes, to temporarily halt ptosis. Also helpful are an abnormal single-giver EMG and/or a decremental response to repetitive nerve stimulation. Immunosuppressants are often prescribed, and anticholinesterase drugs relieve symptoms. It is possible to cure myasthenia gravis with a resection of thymoma.

Status epilepticus

Status epilepticus is any epileptic seizure that lasts for longer than half an hour. This is a very serious problem that requires immediate treatment. Status epilepticus may be caused by anoxic brain injury, trauma, infection, or a withdrawal from anticonvulsants. In order to diagnose the cause of status epilepticus, the patient should be assessed with pulse oximetry, a complete blood count, liver function test, and a toxicology screen. The patient should be fully stabilized before brain imaging and electroencephalography are performed. The patient may require intravenous benzodiazepine and even phenobarbitol. In order to fully stabilize the patient and resolve any unknown deficiencies, glucose, thiamine, and uxalone may be administered.

Alzheimer's disease

Introduction -- Over half of all cases of dementia are caused by Alzheimer's. Dementia of this kind begins slowly and may take a long time to become noticeable. Researchers have outlined three stages in dementia of the Alzheimer's Type. In the first stage, which usually comprises the first one to three years of the condition, the individual suffers from mild anterograde amnesia, especially for declarative memories. He or she is likely to have diminished visuospatial skill, which often manifests itself in wandering aimlessly. Also common to this stage are indifference; irritability; sadness, and anomia. In the second stage, which can stretch between the second and tenth years of the illness, the individual suffers increasing retrograde amnesia; restlessness, delusions, aphasia, acalculia, ideomotor apraxia (the inability to translate an idea into movement), and a generally flat mood.

Symptoms -- In the third stage of Alzheimer's disease, the individual suffers severely impaired intellectual functioning; apathy; limb rigidity; and urinary and fecal incontinence. This last stage usually occurs between the eighth and twelfth years of the condition. Alzheimer's disease is quite difficult to diagnose directly, so it is usually only diagnosed once all the other possible causes of dementia have been eliminated. A brain biopsy that indicates extensive neuron loss, amyloid plaques, and neurofibrillary tangles can give solid evidence of Alzheimer's disease. Individuals who develop Alzheimer's disease usually only live about ten years after onset. The disease is more common in females than males, and is more likely to occur after the age of 65.

Etiology and treatment -- Particular kinds of Alzheimer's disease have been linked with specific genetic abnormalities. For instance, early-onset familial Alzheimer's victims often have abnormalities on chromosome 21, while individuals whose onset is later are likely to have irregularities on chromosome 19. Victims of Alzheimer's disease have also been shown to have significant aluminum deposits in brain tissues, a malfunctioning immune system, and a low level of acetylcholine. Some of the drugs used to treat Alzheimer's increase the cholinergic activity in the brain. These drugs, which include the trade names Cognex and Aricept, can temporarily reverse cognitive impairment, though these improvements are not sustained when the drugs are removed.

Though Alzheimer's disease is a degenerative condition with no known cure, there are a number of different treatments that can provide help to those who suffer from the disease. Group therapy has been found useful, especially when it focuses on orienting the individual in reality and encouraging him or her to reminisce about past experience. Oftentimes, the depression that accompanies Alzheimer's can be alleviated with antidepressant medication. Patients may benefit from vitamin E. Both behavioral techniques and antipsychotic drugs are used to fight the agitation associated with Alzheimer's, and both environmental manipulation and pharmacotherapy have been successful at improving memory and cognitive function.

Vascular dementia

In order to be diagnosed with vascular dementia, an individual must have cognitive impairment and either focal neurological signs or laboratory evidence of cerebrovascular disease. Focal neurological signs may include exaggerated reflexes, weaknesses in the extremities, and abnormalities in gait. Vascular dementia can have varying symptoms, depending on where the brain damage lies. It also tends to progress with gradually increasing severity. Individuals are at particular risk for vascular dementia if they have hypertension, diabetes, are a cigarette smoker, or have atrial fibrillation. In some cases, an individual may be able to recover from vascular dementia; stroke victims, for instance, will notice a great deal of improvement in the first six months after the cerebrovascular accident. Most of this improvement will be in the physical rather than the cognitive symptoms.

Huntington's disease

Individuals with Huntington's disease suffer degeneration of the GABA-producing cells in the substantia nigra, basal ganglia, and cortex. This inherited disease typically appears between the ages of 30 and 40. The affective symptoms of Huntington's disease include irritability, depression, and/or apathy. After a while, the individual will begin to display cognitive symptoms as well, including forgetfulness and dementia. Later, motor symptoms will emerge, including fidgeting, clumsiness, athetosis (slow, writhing movements), and chorea (involuntary quick jerks). Because the affective symptoms appear in advance of the cognitive and motor symptoms, many Huntington's victims are misdiagnosed with depression. Individuals in the early stages of Huntington's may be at risk of suicide, as they will be aware of their impending deterioration and will have the loss of impulse control associated with the disease. Huntington's disease is typically treated with haloperidol for the psychotic symptoms.

Lambert-Eaton myasthenic syndrome

Lambert-Eaton myasthenic syndrome consists of a patient suffering from weakness and exhaustion of the proximal muscles and depressed or absent DTRs. The primary risk factor is small cell lung carcinoma, which is present in 90% of cases. To diagnose this disorder, perform a chest CT to look for lung neoplasm, and look for autoantibodies in presynaptic calcium channels. It is possible for symptoms to be treated or reversed through tumor resection, but guanidine hydrochloride is the primary form of way to manage Lambert-Eaten myasthenic syndrome. Anticholinesterases, which are helpful in other neuromuscular disorders, are also a way for the symptoms to be controlled.

Parkinson's disease

The following symptoms are commonly associated with Parkinson's disease: bradykinesia (general slowness of movement); resting tremor; stoic and unmoving facial expression; loss of coordination and/or balance; an involuntary movement of the thumb and forefinger that resembles rolling a pill; and akathesia (violent restlessness). Most Parkinson's victims will suffer from depression at some point during their illness, and between 20 and 60% will develop dementia. Research has indicated that Parkinson's victims have a deficiency of dopamine-producing cells and the presence of Lewy bodies in the substantia nigra. Many doctors now believe that there is some environmental cause for Parkinson's, though the etiology is not yet clear. The medication L-dopa has famously been shown to alleviate the symptoms of Parkinson's by increasing the amount of dopamine in the brain. Severe cases may benefit from surgical pallidotomy or chronic deep brain stimulation.

Multiple sclerosis

Introduction and symptoms -- This disease is the result of a loss myelin. Myelin coats nerve fibers, allowing nerve fiber conduction. Its decrease can lead to nerve cell death, and causes impaired bodily functions. While is not known what exactly causes multiple sclerosis, the etiology might be autoimmune or vital, both of which are believed to be T-cell mediated. Most patients are diagnosed between the ages of 20 and 40, and the female to male ratio is 3:2. Subtypes are relapsing/remitting, secondary progressive, and primary progressive. The majority of patients experience progressive symptoms, though some enter periods (sometimes permanent) remission. Among the symptoms are limb weakness, optic neuritis, paresthesias, diplopia, urinary retention, vertigo, and paralysis. There are multiple neurologic complaints occurring at different times and parts of the body that are not the result of a single lesion. While attacks are unpredictable, they typically occur every 1.5 years and last for 6 to 8 weeks.

Diagnosis and treatment -- To diagnose MS, an MRI can reveal multiple, asymmetric, and often periventricular white matter lesions (known as Dawson's fingers), often in the corpus callosum. Test cerebrospinal fluid for mononuclear pleocytosis (less than 5 cells/microL), an increased IgC index, or oligoclonal bands. There is no cure for MS, though some symptoms (such as depression, fagitue, and vergito) may be treated, and it is often recommended that lifestyle changes to reduce stress or triggers be made. Steroids are given during acute exacerbations. Immunomodulators will alter relapse rates for relapsing/remitting MS, and mitoxantrone can be given for if relapsing/remitting MS gets worse or for progressive MS.

Amyotrophic Lateral Sclerosis (ALS)

Also known as Lou Gehrig's disease, amyotrophic lateral sclerosis is a progressive, chronic, degenerative disease in whch the upper and lower motor neurons are lost. It happens most often to patients over 50. Most patients die within 2 to 7 years, due to respiratory failure or other diseases that attack as the body weakens. The patient may present with fascillations, and all will have slowly progressive weakening of the arms, legs, and cranial nerves. Patient may also have UMN and/or LMN signs. Though symptoms usually diagnose, an EMG/nerve conduction study can show widespread denervation and fibrillation potentials. There is no cure for ALS, nor is its cause known. Treatment consists of supporting and educating patient and patient's family.

Guillain-Barre Syndrome (GBS)

This autoimmune disorder consists of acute, rapidly progressive demyelination of the peripheral nerves (often beginning in legs) that leads to weakness. It is associated with viral infections and influenza vaccination. The vast majority of patients make a complete or near-complete recovery, though it may take up to a year. There is a mortality rate of less than 5%. Patient may present with quickly worsening ascending paralysis of the trunk, diaphragm, and cranial nerves. There can also be autonomic symptoms, hyporeflexia, areflexia, and dysesthesias. To diagnose, look for diffuse demyelination on EMG and perform nerve conduction studies. A CSF protein level of below 55 mg/dL is also common. Admit patient to the ICU due to risk of respiratory failure, and treat with plasmapheresis and IVIG—not steroids. It is absolutely necessary to pursue aggressive physical rehabilitation.

Neoplasms

Introduction and symptoms -- Neoplasms, also known as tumors, occur in different parts of the body and have varying symptoms. The symptoms occur as a result of the location and type of tumor, the local growth and its resulting mass effect, ventricular obstruction, cerebral edema, and increased ICP. Some symptoms, which develop over time, include nausea, vomiting, headaches, focal neurologic deficits, and possible lethary, asphasias, mood swings, lethargy, seizures, and intellectual decline. Intracranial neoplasms are either 1st degree (30%) or metastatic (70%). 40% of 1st degree brain tumors and these usually do not spread past the CNS. Melanoma and 1st degree lung, breast, kidney, and GI tract neoplasms usually result in metastatic intracranial tumors, which happen at the gray-white junction and might occur in multiple discrete nodules.

Diagnosis and treatment -- To diagnose neoplasms, contract CT and MRI with gadolinium in order to localize and use a CT-guided biopsy or surgical tumor debulking for histology. Treatment options are resection if possible, radiation, and chemotheraphy. The different types of treatment are applied to tumors according to their location, type, histology, and progression. To reduce vasogenic edema, prescribe corticosteroids. Treatment is often palliative, since there are some tumors (such as grade IV astrocytoma) with an incredibly poor prognosis. Others simply cannot be resected, and so symptoms resulting from chemotheraphy and/or radiation should be treated.

Neurofibromatosis (NF)

Introduction -- The most common neurocutaneous disorder, neurofibromatosis has two different forms: NF1 (also known as von Recklinghausen's disease) and NF2. It is a genetic disorder of the nervous system that affects neural cell tissues. NF1 is inherited in an autosomal dominant manner and is the result of a mutation on the NF1 gene (in chromosome band 17q11) which encodes the protein neurofibromin. NF2 is also inherited in an autosomal dominant manner, but is caused by a mutation in the NF2 gene (in chromosome band 22q12.2), which encodes the protein merlin. Around 50% of cases are due to new mutations of each gene, and prenatal testing is available to detect both NF1 and NF2.

Diagnosis and treatment -- To diagnose NF1, patients must present with two or more of the following: six café-au-lait spots, freckling in the axillary or inguinal area, two of any type of neurofibromas, optic glioma, bone abnormality, two Lisch nodules, or a first-degree relative with NF1. To diagnose NF2, look for bilateral acoustic neuromas or a first-degree relative with NF2 *and* unilateral acoustic neuromas *or* any two of the following: neurofibromas, meningiomas, gliomas, or schwannoma. Patient may also have café-au-lait spots, skin nodules, and seizures. Perform an MRI of the brain, brain stem, and spine, and perform a complete dermatological exam, ophthalmologic exam, and get the family history. It is also suggested to perform auditory testing. NF1 and NF2 are incurable, but symptoms can be treated. It is also possible to treat acoustic neuromas with surgery or radiosurgery.

Broca's aphasia

In Broca's aphasia, an individual will only be able to speak slowly and with great difficulty. Individuals with this form of aphasia will often suffer from anomia, the inability to name familiar objects. Broca's aphasia, unlike many impairments, does not include a lack of self-awareness, so individuals are likely to become very frustrated by their deficits and impairments. This condition is typically caused by injury to the posterior inferior frontal gyrus, and is often preceded by a left superior MCA stroke. Individuals with this condition, which is also known as expressive or nonfluent aphasia, should be given speech therapy, even though this treatment has a spotty record of success.

Tuberous Sclerosis

Tuberous sclerosis is a genetic disease that affects the skin, brain, kidneys, and heart. There are always skin abnormalities, among them "ash-leaf" hypopigmented lesions on the trunk and extremities, sebaceous adenomas, and a shagreen patch. A patient may also suffer infantile spasms and mental retardation, the likelihood of which increases with an early age of tuberous sclerosis's onset. There are two retinal lesions: mulberry tumors, arising from the nervehead, and phakomas, which are round, flat, gray lesions near the optic disk. The patient may also suffer angiomyolipomas, rhabdomyomas, and arrhythmias. To diagnose, perform a head CT to look for calcified tubers in the periventricular area. The patient's skin lesions can be seen under an ultraviolet light, and a renal ultrasound might indicate renal hamartomas or plycystic disease. Also get an ECG to look for rhabdomyoma of the heart. The symptoms can be treated, especially seizures, and surgery might be necessary for increased intracranial pressure.

Coma

A coma is a profound lack of response to any internal or external stimuli. Coma can be caused by a number of different things, but it is most often caused by head trauma, poisoning, or disease. In order to fully assess a comatose patient, a doctor should obtain a complete medical history, and should perform an examination that includes mental status, papillary response, cold-water calorics, and response to noxious stimuli (i.e., smelling salts). An electroencephalogram is often performed on comatose patients, and to differentiate between alpha, spindle, and theta comas. An examination should seek to differentiate coma from persistent vegetative state. The treatment for comatose patients includes stabilization, administering dextrose, oxygen, naloxone, and thiamine, and attempting to treat the underlying cause of the coma.

Aphasia

Wernicke's aphasia -- Caused by damage to the left temporal lobe. It is characterized by difficulty understanding and generating meaningful language. People with this condition will be capable of talking quite fluently, but will be unable to say anything consequential.

Conduction aphasia -- A condition that includes anomia and impaired repetition.

Transcortical aphasia -- Caused by lesions that disconnect Broca's and Wernicke's areas from other parts of the brain. If Broca's area is isolated, then the individual way labor to speak, may be unable to speak spontaneously, and may suffer from anomia. If Wernicke's area is isolated, the individual may have deficits in comprehension, anomia, and fluent but meaningless speech. The patient should be given speech therapy, though the prognosis is not great.

Glaucoma

Open-angle glaucoma -- Open-angle glaucoma is more common than closed-angle glaucoma. In this condition, the fluid pressure in the eye increases markedly because of diminished drainage from the eye. Individuals are at special risk of open-angle glaucoma if they are over 40 years old and African-American. Patients with this condition will often present with mild headaches and a frequent need to change corrective lenses. As the condition deteriorates, individuals will often notice that their peripheral vision is poor. A positive diagnosis of open-angle glaucoma can be obtained by tonometry and an opthalmascopic visualization of the optic nerve. Patients with open-angle glaucoma typically also have a diseased trabecular meshwork. Patients may be treated with topical beta-blockers or pilocarpine; as a last resort, laser trabeculoplasty may be performed

Closed-angle glaucoma -- Closed-angle glaucoma is an increase in the pressure of the anterior chamber of the eye that is caused by an obstruction in the normal circulation of the eye's fluid.

Individuals are more likely to develop this kind of glaucoma as they grow older, and if they are undergoing papillary dilation for a long period. The symptoms of closed-angle glaucoma are severe eye and facial pain, vomiting and nausea, the perception of a halo around any lights, and blurred vision. This condition needs to be treated immediately, as it can result in optic nerve damage and subsequent vision loss. The pressure within the eye can be diminished with acetazolamide followed by pilocarpine; a more permanent cure is provided by laser iridotomy.

Macular degeneration

Macular degeneration is the deterioration of the macula lutea, which can result in diminished fine frontal vision. This condition is especially common among females, Caucasians, and smokers, and seems to be an inherited disorder. Patients with macular degeneration present with a painless loss of their central vision. There are two kinds of macular degeneration, known as the dry and wet types. The wet type is far more common, and first appears as the perception of straight lines as wavy. In dry macular degeneration, the decrease in frontal vision is slower. A positive diagnosis of macular degeneration can be made after a fundoscopy indicates a pigmentary or hemorrhagic problem. Treatment is difficult, though some wet cases may benefit from laser photocoagulation.

Cardiovascular Disorders

Normal electrocardiogram

The normal heart rate is between 60 and 10 beats per minute. Anything lower is bradyarrhtyhmia; anything higher is tachyarrhythmia. When looking at an electrocardiogram, the doctor should check for a sinus rhythm; that is, a P before every QRS and a QRS after every P. Also, the doctor should check for any irregular rhythms, and juctional or ventricular rhythms (when there is no P before a QRS). A normal axis will have upright QRS in leads I and aVF. If there is an upright QRS in lead I and a downward QRS in lead aVF, this is a left-axis deviation. If there is a downward QRS in lead I and an upright QRS in lead aVF, this is a right-axis deviation. As for intervals, when checking an ECG a doctor should be looking for heart block, in which there is a PR interval of more than 2 msec or a P with no successive QRS, or bundle branch blocks (QRS of greater than 120 msec).

Bradyarrhythmias

Left bundle branch block (LBBB) -- Usually a sign of organic heart disease, as for instance hypertension, valvular disease, cardiomyopathy, and CAD. It is typically asymptomatic, and requires no treatment (though it may be resolved via pacemaker). On an ECG, LBBB appears as QRS with duration greater than 120 msec; a wide, negative QS complex in V; and a broad, tall R wave with no Q wave in V sub-6.

First-degree AV block is also asymptomatic and requires no treatment; its ECG features a PR interval greater than 200 msec. First-degree AV block is associated with elevated vagal tone as well as with beta blockers and calcium channel blockers.
Second-degree AV block, also known as Mobitz I -- Can be caused by certain drugs (digoxin, beta blockers, calcium channel blockers) and by increased vagal tone. It usually has no symptoms, and is represented on an ECG as elevated PR interval until a dropped beat occurs, at which point the PR resets. When this occurs as a result of a medication, use of the medication should be suspended immediately.

Sinus bradycardia -- Can result from sinus node dysfunction or from an excess of beta blockers or calcium channel blockers. Though it is often asymptomatic, it may occur with light-headedness, syncope, and hypotension. On the ECG, the ventricular rate will be less than 60 bpm, and there will be normal P waves before every QRS complex. Sinus bradycardia does not need to be treated if it is asymptomatic, though atropine is often used to raise the heart rate. The condition may be fully resolved with a pacemaker.

There is also no treatment necessary for Right Bundle Branch Block (RBBB), a condition which may result from COPD, valvular disease, or chronic CAD, or may follow the surgical repair of VSD. There are no symptoms, and the ECG will display a QRS greater than 120 msec in duration, with rSR complexes with a wide R wave in V sub-1 and a QRS with a wide S wave in V sub-6.

The variety of second-degree AV block known as Mobitz II is caused by fibrotic disease of the conduction system or by a previous septal MI. Symptoms may include syncope or progression to third-degree AV block. On an ECG, it appears as an unexpected dropped beat without a change in PR interval. The only solution to this problem is pacemaker placement.

Third-degree, or complete AV block, is the result of there being absolutely no electrical communication between the atria and ventricles. Symptoms include syncope, dizziness, acute heart failure, hypotension, and cannon A waves. On the ECG, it will appear that there is no relationship between the P waves and QRS complexes. Again, the only solution is the placement of a pacemaker.

Supraventricular tachyarrhythmias

Sinus tachycardia is an elevated heart rate and is a normal response to fear, exercise, and pain. It may also be caused by hyperthyroidism, dehydration, infection, or a pulmonary embolism. Symptoms of sinus tachycardia include palpitations and shortness of breath; the condition appears on the ECG as a ventricular rate greater than 100 bpm with normal P waves before every QRS complex. The condition does not require treatment, though the underlying condition may.

The etiology of atrial fibrillation can be remembered using the mnemonic PIRATES: Pulmonary disease, Ischemia, Rheumatic heart disease, Anemia/Atrial myxoma, Thyrotoxicosis, Ethanol, Sepsis. Though it is often asymptomatic, the condition may present with shortness of breath, chest pain, palpitations, and irregularly irregular pulse. On an ECG, it will appear as a wavy baseline without discernible P waves, with a variable and irregular QRS response. Treatment may include anticoagulation (to prevent stroke) and rate control, which may be accomplished with beta or calcium channel blockers. Cardioversion is necessary only when new onset occurs within 48 hours.

Atrioventricular reciprocating tachycardia (AVRT) is caused by the circular movement of an impulse down the AV node and back up the atrium through a bypass tract. This condition, which is seen in Wolff-Parkinson-White syndrome, may be characterized by palpitations, shortness of breath, angina, syncope, and light-headedness. On the ECG, the retrograde P wave will frequently appear after a normal QRS wave. Treatment for AVRT is the same as for AVNRT.

Paroxysmal atrial tachycardia is caused by a rapid ectopic pacemaker in the atrium, not the sinus node. The symptoms of this condition include palpitations, shortness of breath, angina, syncope, and light-headedness. On the ECG, paroxysmal atrial tachycardia appears as a ventricular rate greater than 100 bpm, and a P wave with an unusual axis before each normal QRS. As for treatment, adenosine may be used in order to diagnose the condition.

Atrial flutter is caused by a circular movement of the electrical activity at a rate of 300 times a minute. It is usually asymptomatic, though it may appear with palpitations, syncope, and light-headedness. On the ECG, it will appear as a regular rhythm with sawtooth appearance of P waves. Treatment includes anticoagulation and rate control. Cardioversion is only necessary when new onset occurs within 48 hours.

Multifocal atrial tachycardia is asymptomatic and is caused by multiple atrial pacemakers or reentrant pathways, COPD, or hypoxemia. An ECG will appear as three or more unique P-wave morphologies, with a ventricular rate of more than 100 bpm. Treatment should be concerned with the underlying causes, and should include verapamil or beta blockers for rate control and the suppression of the atrial pacemakers.

Atrial nodal reentry tachycardia (AVNRT) occurs when a reentry circuit in the AV node depolarizes the atrium and ventricle simultaneously. Symptoms include palpitations, shortness of breath, angina, syncope, and light-headedness. On the ECG, the ventricular rate will be 150-250 bpm; P wave may be buried within QRS or directly after. Treatment may include carotid massage, Valsalva, or adenosine to stop the arrhythmia. Cardioversion may be necessary if the person becomes hemodynamically unstable.

Ventricular tachyarrhythmias

One common form of ventricular tachyarrhythmia is ventricular tachycardia. Ventricular tachycardia, which is associated with CAD and MI, may be asymptomatic if it is not sustained. If it is sustained, however, it may lead to palpitations, hypotension, angina, and syncope. Eventually, the condition may lead to ventricular fibrillation. On the ECG, the condition will appear as three or more consecutive PVCs, with wide QRS complexes in a regular rapid rhythm. Also, there may be some AV dissociation, in which there will be no discernible P waves. Treatment for the condition should include cardioversion and the administration of antiarrhythmics, which may include amiodarone, lidocaine, and procainamide.

Premature ventricular contractions caused by ectopic beats arising from the ventricular foci. This condition, which is associated with hypoxia, electrolyte abnormalities, and hyperthyroidism, is often without symptoms, but may lead to palpitations. The ECG will display an early, broad QRS that is not preceded by a P wave; PVCs will be followed by a compensatory pause. Treatment should be concerned with the underlying cause; if the condition is symptomatic, the patient should be given beta blockers or other antiarrhythmics.

Ventricular fibrillation is a condition associated with CAD and MI; symptoms may include syncope, hypotension, and lack of a pulse. On the ECG, ventricular fibrillation will appear as totally erratic tracing. Treatment should include immediate electrical cardioversion and the ACLS protocol.

Dilated cardiomyopathy

In order for a diagnosis of dilated cardiomyopathy to be made, left ventricular dilation and systolic function must be present. Though most instances of this condition are idiopathic: the following may also contribute: alcohol, wet beriberi, cossackievirus, Chagas' disease, parasites, cocaine, myocarditis, doxorubicin, HIV, and AZT use. Second-degree dilated cardiomyopathy is often caused by ischemia and long-standing hypertension. The condition usually begins with the gradual development of symptoms similar to those of congestive heart failure. The examination will often require cardiomegaly and an S3 in addition to tricuspid and mitral regurgitation. In order to diagnose the condition, echocardiography can be used. The ECG of someone with this condition may show nonspecific ST-T changes, low-voltage QRS, sinus tachycardia, and ectopy. Left bundle branch block may appear. The chest X-ray will display a large, balloon-shaped heart and pulmonary congestion.

ECG abnormalities

A ventricular hypertrophy is diagnosed as LVH when the amplitude of the R wave in aVL plus the amplitude of the S wave in the V sub-3 is greater than or equal to 24 mm for males or greater than 20 mm in females. A ventricular hypertrophy is diagnosed as RVH when there is right-axis deviation and the R wave in V sub-1 is greater than 7 mm. Atrial hypertrophy is diagnosed as right atrial enlargement if the P wave amplitude in lead II is greater than 2.5 mm; it is diagnosed as left atrial enlargement if there is a biphasic P wave in lead V sub-1. Hyperkalemia features peaked T waves, a widening of the PR interval, a widening of QRS, and a sinusoidal wave pattern that may lead to ventricular fibrillation. Pulmonary embolus appears on an ECG as sinus tachycardia, S wave in lead I, Q wave in lead III, and an inverted T wave in lead III. Wolff-Parkinson-White syndrome occurs when an electrical charge excites the ventricle prematurely after bypassing the AV node; this causes the ECG to show a delta wave before QRS. This condition can lead to fatal AVRT.

Congestive heart failure

American Heart Association classification and treatment of congestive heart failure -- In stage A, the patient is at a high risk of developing congestive heart failure due to the presence of risk factors, but there is no identified structural or functional abnormality, and there are no signs or symptoms of CHF. In this stage, the patient should try to manage his or her treatable risk factors. In stage B, the patient may be given angiotensin-converting enzyme inhibitors (ACEIs) or beta-blockers, as they will have structural heart disease without any symptoms of congestive heart failure. Stage C contains those patients who have structural heart disease and have had previous or current symptoms of congestive heart failure. Treatment for these patients may include diuretics, ACEIs, beta-blockers, digitalis, and dietary salt restriction. Stage D contains those patients who have marked symptoms of congestive heart failure at rest despite total medical therapy. For these patients, treatment may include mechanical assist devices, heart transplant, continuous IV inotropic drugs, and hospice care.

Congestive heart failure is the clinical presentation of cardiomyopathy. Congestive heart failure is likely to ensue when the patient's heart is unable to fulfill the requirements of oxygen of the heart and the body tissues. There are a few risk factors associated with congestive heart failure: coronary artery disease, hypertension, valvular heart disease, pericardial disease, cardiomyopathy, and pulmonary hypertension. The common causes of recurrent congestive heart failure can be remembered using the mnemonic FAILURE: Forgot medication, Arrhythmia/Anemia, Ischemia/Infarct/Infection, Lifestyle (for instance, little or no exercise), Upregulation (increased cardiac output), and embolus.

Systolic dysfunction -- An individual with the form of congestive heart failure known as systolic dysfunction has an ejection fraction less than 50%. This condition is caused by diminished contractile function in the left ventricle. The decreased ejection fraction leads to an increase in preload, with an accompanying increase in left ventricular end-diastolic pressure. The problem culminates in increased systolic contractility according to the Frank-Starling law. The heart may try to compensate for this problem, but this will eventually cause hypertrophy, ventricular dilation, and increased myocardial work. A patient with systolic dysfunction will typically complain of dyspnea during exertion or, in severe cases, while at rest. Patients may also have chronic cough, fatigue, lower extremity edema, orthopnea, paroxysmal nocturnal dyspnea, and/or abdominal fullness.

The chest X-ray of a patient with systolic dysfunction will show evidence of cardiomegaly, cephalization of pulmonary vessels, pleural effusions, vascular indistinctness, and prominent hila. The echocardiogram will display impaired cardiac function, while the ECG may indicate atrial fibrillation. If the condition is acute, it may need to be distinguished from myocardial infarction. In acute cases, the underlying causes should be treated and the patient should be administered a loop diuretic and a non-loop diuretic. Also, potassium levels should be monitored with potassium-sparing agents. Unless they are intolerable, ACEIs should be administered; beta-blockers should not be administered during decompensated congestive heart failure.

Chronic cases of congestive heart failure should be treated with long-term beta-blockers and ACEIs/angiotensin receptor blockers in order to prevent the neurohormonal remodeling of the heart. Patients should also take a daily Aspirin and a statin to discourage further ischemic events. Diuretic therapy is often provided to prevent volume overload. Patients with left ventricular systolic dysfunction and NYHA class III or IV heart failure are often given low-dose spironolactone in combination with ACEIs and loop diuretics to reduce the risk of death. Arrhythmias must be treated if they arise, and dietary sodium and fluid intake should be controlled. Patients with severe dilated cardiomyopathy, atrila fibrillation, or previous embolic episodes may need warfarin. If a congestive heart failure patient is resistant to treatment, cardiac transplantation or a mechanical left ventricular assist device may be necessary.

Diastolic dysfunction -- The form of congestive heart failure known as diastolic dysfunction characterized by decreased ventricular compliance with normal contractile function. In this condition, the ventricle is either unable to relax or to passively fill in the proper manner. The heart manifests increased stiffness, decreased recoil, and concentric hypertrophy. There will be an increase in left ventricular-enddiastoluc pressure, while cardiac output will remain average and ejection fraction will be about average or slightly elevated. Patients with diastolic dysfunction will have stable and unstable angina, shortness of breath, dyspnea upon exertion, arrhythmias, myocardial infarction, heart failure, and sudden death. Treatment typically includes beta-blockers, ACEIs, diuretics, rate control, blood pressure management. Patients with this condition should not be given Digoxin.

Coronary artery disease

Angina pectoris -- Characterized by substernal chest pain due to myocardial ischemia, resulting in either an elevated oxygen demand or a diminished oxygen supply. The so-called triad of angina pectoris is substernal chest pain which is aggravated by exertion and relieved by both rest and nitrates. This pain may radiate to the arms, jaw, and neck, and can often lead to nausea, light-headedness, or shortness of breath. An ECG may indicate ST-segment depression or T-wave flattening. The acute symptoms of angina pectoris can be treated with morphine, oxygen, sublingual nitroglycerine, ASA and IV beta-blockers. Patients who may have a myocardial infacrction will need to be admitted into a hospital and treated until serial cardiac enzymes can rule out acute myocardial infarction. Chronic symptoms may be treated with nitrates, beta-blockers, and calcium channel blockers. The various risk factors (e.g. smoking, hypertension) must also be considered.

Hypercholesterolemia -- The clinical manifestations of coronary artery disease include stable and unstable angina, shortness of breath, dyspnea on exertion, arrhythmias, myocardial infarction, heart failure, and sudden death. The variety of CAD known as hypercholesterolemia is associated with elevated blood cholesterol, increased low-density lipoprotein, increased triglycerides, and decreased high-density lipoproteins. It is caused by obesity, Cushing's disease, alcoholism, and hyperthyroidisms, among other things. Most patients with hypercholesterolemia have no signs or symptoms, though those patients with extremely high triglycerides or low-density lipoproteins may develop xanthomas, xanthelasmas, and lipemia retinalis. This condition is diagnosed by means of a fasting lipid profile for patients over twenty years old; if the individual has total serum cholesterol greater than 200 mg/dL, LDL greater than 130 mg/dL, or HDL less than 35 mg/dL, then hypercholesterolemia may be diagnosed. Treatment begins with adjustments in diet and exercise.

Unstable angina -- The variety of coronary artery disease known as unstable angina is diagnosed if angina is new, accelerating, or occurs while the patient is at rest. Angina is considered to be accelerating if it occurs with less exertion, lasts for a longer period, and is less responsive to medications. Unstable angina may indicate a transient vessel occlusion; in other words, the interruption of blood flow caused by an atherosclerotic plaque and/or vasoplasm in the area of the plaque. Unstable angina may also indicate an area of myocardial ischemia that has the potential to lead to myocardial infarction or complete occlusion. As for treatment, acute unstable angina is typically treated in the same manner as stable angina, though the glycoprotein IIB-IIIA inhibitors may be used. Treatment may also include heparinization, angiography, and possible revascularization.

Myocardial infarction

Introduction and symptoms -- Myocardial infarction is typically caused by an occlusive thrombus or an extended vasospasm in a coronary artery. These are most frequently the result of acute thrombus on a ruptured atherosclerotic plaque. Patients suffering from MI will complain of acute-onset substernal chest pain, which feels like a pressure or tightness and can radiate to the left arm, neck, and jaw. Some patients may develop diaphoresis, shortness of breath, lightheadedness, anxiety, and syncope. The examining doctor should look for tachycardia, bradycardia, arrhythmia, new mitral regurgitation, hypotension, rales, and ventricular fibrillation. One-fifth of all those who suffer from MI will die suddenly as a result of a lethal arrhythmia. Some patients, especially those who are elderly, diabetic, or postmenopausal, may present with no discernible symptoms.

Diagnosis and treatment -- Myocardial infarction often is indicated on an ECG by ST-segment elevations or new LBBB. Changes in the patient's ECG will proceed in the following sequence: peaked T waves, ST-segment elevation, Q waves, T wave inversion, ST segment normalization, T wave normalization. The elevation in the ST segment in II, III, and aVF are consistent with inferior MI. If the elevations are in the anterior leads, this indicates anterior MI; elevations in leads I, aVL, and V sub-5/sub-6 indicate lateral MI. Treatment for MI is the same as for unstable angina, though it may be necessary to consider emergent angiography and revascularization, or even thrombolysis with tPA, urokinase, or streptokinase. When there is a single or double vessel disease with discrete lesions, the patient may require PTCA. Complications may include Dressler's syndrome, an autoimmune process with fever, pericarditis, pleura effusion, leukocytosis, and elevated ESR.

First degree (essential) hypertension

Hypertension is defined as blood pressure greater than 140 and/or a diastolic blood pressure greater than 90. These figures must be confirmed by three measures taken over the course of two weeks. First degree hypertension is associated with a family history of hypertension, a high-sodium diet, smoking, obesity, and advanced age. Typically, elevated blood pressure will be asymptomatic until complications develop. If left untreated, first degree hypertension may lead to heart, kidney, and eye damage. Before it can be treated, first degree hypertension must be distinguished from second degree hypertension. Patients should try to improve their diet and exercise habits. For otherwise healthy patients, the goal of treatment should be blood pressure less than 140 with a diastolic less than 90. For patients with uncomplicated hypertension, diuretics and beta blockers have been shown to reduce the chances of sudden fatality.

Hypertensive urgency

Hypertensive urgency is clinically defined as blood pressure greater than 180 (diastolic greater than 130) that is asymptomatic or moderately symptomatic. A hypertensive emergency, on the other hand, may occur at any blood pressure, but is defined as signs or symptoms of impending end-organ damage, such as acute renal failure or hematuria. Other symptoms include altered mental status due to neurological disease, intercranial hemorrhage, papilledema, vascular changes, and pulmonary edema. Malignant hypertension is progressive renal failure and/or encephalopathy with papilledema. The diagnosis of these conditions is typically made after cardiovascular, neurologic, ophthalmologic, and abdominal exams. The patient's blood pressure must be diminished slowly, in order to prevent cerebral hypofusion or coronary insufficiency. Beta blockers, ACEIs, and clonidine are preferable to calcium channel blockers.

Second degree hypertension

Second degree hypertension is caused by some identifiable organic cause. If it is caused by first degree renal disease, it should be treated with ACEIs. If it is caused by renal artery stenosis, it should be treated with angioplasty and stenting if possible. If it is the result of Conn's or Cushing's syndromes, the problematic tumor should be removed surgically. For women over the age of 35 or obese women, second degree hypertension may be caused by the use of oral contraceptives. In this case, treatment generally just consists of discontinuing the use of the OCP. If the cause of hypertension is coarctation of the aorta, then surgical repair may be necessary.

Cardiac tamponade

Cardiac tamponade is characterized by an excess of fluid in the pericardial sac that leads to impaired filling of the ventricles and a decreased cardiac output. This condition is more closely tied to the rate of fluid formation than with the size of the effusion. Risk factors for cardiac tamponade are pericarditis, malignancy, tuberculosis, and trauma. A patient with this condition will typically present with fatigue, dyspnea, tachycardia, and tachypnea. This last condition can quickly result in shock and death. An echocardiogram will often indicate right atrial and right ventricular diastolic collapse, while the chest X-ray will indicate an enlarged, globular heart. Treatment for this condition includes an aggressive volume expansion with IV fluids as well as urgent pericardiocentesis.

Pericarditis

Pericardial disease typically results from an acute or chronic pericardial insult; this condition can lead in some cases to percicardial effusion. One variety of pericardial disease, known as pericarditis, is characterized by an inflammation of the pericardial sac. This condition can obstruct the output of the heart by tamponade or constrictive pericarditis. Patients with this condition may present with pleuritic chest pain, dyspnea, cough, and fever. The chest pain reported may be positional in nature, meaning that it is worst in the supine position but improves when the patient leans forward. In order to diagnose pericarditis, a chest X ray, ECG, and echocardiogram must be performed in order to differentiate from myocardial infarction and pneumonia. The ECG will likely display PR segment depressions in precordial leads, low voltage, and diffuse ST segment elevation. Treatment should be directed at the underlying cause, though tamponade or large effusions will require pericardiocentosis with continuous drainage.

Mitral valve disease

Mitral stenosis is associated with rheumatic heart disease, and has the same symptoms as congestive heart failure. This condition causes a mid-diastolic rumble with an opening snap at the apex. A physical exam will indicate atrial fibrillation, pulmonary rales, and a right ventricular heave. Treatment for this condition entails avoiding the use of inotropic agents; the administration of beta blockers and diuretics may be recommended. Mitral regurgitation is associated with rheumatic heart disease, myocardial infarction, infective endocarditis, and severe mitral valve prolapse. This is left side heart failure that has the potential to lead to right side heart failure. It has a distinctive murmur: a high-pitched, holosystolic murmur at the apex that radiates to the axilla. Treatment should include ACEIs, vasodilators, and diuretics. Mitral valve prolapse, is typically benign, and occurs in about 7% of the population. A characteristic of this condition is a late systolic murmur with a midsystolic click. No treatment is necessary unless the condition is symptomatic.

Aortic valve disease

Aortic stenosis is associated with rheumatic heart disease, congenital aortic stenosis, and bicuspid valve. The symptoms are the classic triad of exertional dyspnea, angina, and syncope. There will typically be a midsystolic crescendo-decrescendo murmur that is easiest to hear at the second intercostals space, and which radiates to the neck. Physical exam will reveal pulvus parvis et tardis. Treatment for aortic stenosis includes avoiding afterload reducers. Aortic regurgitation is associated with rheumatic heart disease, syphilis, Marfan's syndrome, and congenital bicuspid valve. It may result in congestive heart failure due to volume overload. There are three murmurs associated with this condition: a high-pitched, blowing diastolic murmur found at the left sternal border, an Austin Flint/low-pitched, mid-diastolic rumble, and a midsystolic murmur at the base. A physical exam will indicate widened pulse pressure and a laterally displaced PMI. The treatment for aortic regurgitation is aortic valve replacement.

Aortic dissection

An aortic dissection is a transverse tear in the intima of a vessel that results in blood entering the media. This in turn creates a false lumen and a hematoma that propagates longitudinally. This condition is most often associated with hypertension, and often occurs above the aortic valve and distal to the left subclavian artery. Patients with this condition will feel a sudden tearing or stabbing sensation in an ascending dissection, and an interscapular back pain in a descending dissection. The patient will typically be hypertensive, and signs of pericarditis and pericardial tamponade are often evident. Treatment for this condition includes decreasing the blood pressure if the patient is hypertensive, and performing surgery if the dissection involves the ascending aorta.

Aortic aneurysm

Aortic aneurysms most frequently occur in patients with atherosclerosis. A large majority of these aneurysms occur below the renal arteries. The condition is usually asymptomatic; risk factors include hypertension, high cholesterol, smoking, and age. A physical examination may reveal pulsatile abdominal mass or abdominal bruits; a ruptured aneurysm can lead to hypotension and severe abdominal pain. In order to track an aneurysm, an abdominal ultrasound may be useful. Treatment for this condition may include monitoring lesions less than 5 cm if the patient is asymptomatic and surgical repair of any larger lesions. If the aneurysms are asymptomatic or ruptured, the patient should have surgery.

Peripheral vascular disease

Peripheral vascular disease is the occlusion of the blood supply to the extremities that is caused by atherosclerotic plaques. The patient will often present with intermittent claudication, though there will be a progression to rest pain and ischemia in the distal aspects of the extremities. The diagnosis of this condition requires the careful palpation of pulses and the auscultation of bruits. A Doppler ultrasound may be useful for identifying stenosis and occlusion. For surgical evaluation, arteriography and digital subtraction angiography are necessary. Peripheral vascular disease is treated by controlling the underlying causes, often through exercise. Symptoms may be improved by aspirin, cilostazol, and thromboxane inhibitors. If these treatments fail, surgery may be necessary.

Deep venous thrombosis

Deep venous thrombosis (DVT) is the formation of clots in the large veins of the extremities or the pelvis. This condition is common in people who have had to remain stationary for a long time, who have incompetent venous valves in the lower extremities, or who have congestive heart failure. A patient with this condition will typically present with unilateral lower extremity pain, erythema, and swelling. A Doppler ultrasound will be required to make the diagnosis of DVT. Treatment includes initial anticoagulation with intravenous heparin, followed by warfarin for between 3 and 6 months. Patients that have contraindications to anticoagulation may need to receive an IVC filter.

Respiratory System Diseases

Systemic sarcoidosis

Systemic sarcoidosis is a disease that causes small lumps in the tissues of the body. The cause of systemic sarcoidosis is unknown. Interestingly, the individuals most commonly afflicted by systemic sarcoidosis are African-American females and Norwegians. Patients with systemic sarcoidosis will commonly present with fever, cough, malaise, weight loss, dyspnea, and arthritis. The symptoms of systemic sarcoidosis are often called to mind using the mnemonic GRUELING: granulomas, rheumatoid arthritis, uveitis, erythema nodosum, lymphadenopathy, interstitial fibrosis, negative TB test, and gammaglobulinemia. A diagnosis of systemic sarcoidosis can be made after a biopsy displays noncaseating granulomas and laboratory tests indicate elevated levels of serum angiotensin-converting enzyme and hypercalcemia. In most cases, the granulomas will clear up spontaneously; if they do not, however, they may leave scars. Patients can be treated with systemic corticosteroids.

Interstitial lung disease

Interstitial lung disease is the most common form of lung disease, in which there is a broadening of the walls of the alveoli causing the brinchii to dilate. This condition can be caused by idiopathic pulmonary fibrosis, granumlomatous disorders, and pneumonoconiosis. A patient with interstitial lung disease will typically present with quick, shallow respiration and pronounced dyspnea during and after exertion. Finally, the patient is likely to have a nonproductive cough. A chest X ray will indicate either a reticular pattern or, in more severe cases, a honeycomb pattern. Laboratory tests will indicate normal levels of forced expiratory volume per second, and diminished levels of total lung capacity, diffusing capacity of carbon monoxide, and forced vital capacity. The patient diagnosed with interstitial lung disease should be given supportive treatment and should avoid the agent that causes the condition.

Asthma

Asthma is a form of obstructive lung disease in which an inflammation in the lungs causes the bronchi to become swollen. This narrows the airways and makes breathing difficult. There may also be hypertrophy of the smooth muscles in the throat. Asthmatic patients will present with shortness of breath, cough, wheezing, and tightness in the chest. The patient may also appear with diminished oxygen saturation. A diagnosis of asthma can be made when measures of arterial blood gas indicate mild hypoxia and respiratory alkalosis. A peak flow test will indicate diminished flow, while a chest X ray is likely to indicate hyperinflation. The treatment for asthma may include changes in life style or medication; the medications used to treat asthma can be remembered with the mnemonic ASTHMA: albuterol, steroids, theophylline, humidified oxygen, magnesium, and antileukotrienes.

Hypersensitivity pneumonitis

Hypersensitivity pneumonitis is an inflammation of the lungs that is caused by exposure to some environmental antigen. Some of the sources of these antigens are moldy hay, sugarcane, air conditioners, compost, feather, grain weevil dust, and bird excreta. A patient with acute hypersensitivity pneumonitis will present with fever, dyspnea, and a cough that began 4-6 hours after exposure to the antigen. Chronic hypersensitivity pneumonitis presents with dyspnea, and fine bilateral rales. A chest X ray may show miliary nodular infiltrate, and possible fibrosis in the upper lobes. The patient should be given steroids for inflammation and instructed to avoid the source of the condition.

Chronic obstructive pulmonary disease

Introduction and symptoms -- Chronic obstructive pulmonary disease (COPD) is the blanket name for any respiratory disorder that repeatedly inhibits airflow through the bronchii. A patient with COPD is usually caused by either chronic bronchitis or emphysema. The etiology is considered to be emphysema if the patient smokes or suffers from an alpha sub-1 antitrypsin deficiency. Unfortunately, this condition often does not become known until more than half of lung function is lost. Patients suffering from COPD as a result of emphysema will present with dyspnea, late hypercarbia or hypoxia, and characteristically puckered lips. Patients suffering from COPD as a result of chronic bronchitis present with a productive cough, wheezing, and early hypercarbia/hypoxia.

Diagnosis and treatment -- Chronic obstructive pulmonary disease can be diagnosed after a chest X ray displays diminished lung markings, hyperinflated lungs, parenchymal blisters, and subpleural blebs. Lung function tests will indicate diminished forced vital capacity and forced expiratory volume. Tests of arterial blood gas will indicate hypoxemia with acute respiratory acidosis. If there is a productive cough, it may be useful to perform a Gram stain or sputum culture. As for treatment, acute cases of COPD can be mitigated with oxygen, beta-agonists, antibiotics, intravenous steroids, and anticholinergics. Chronic cases can be treated with the immediate cessation of smoking, flu vaccines, and supplemental oxygen. COPD cannot be entirely cured.

Bronchiectasis

Bronchiectasis is caused by recurring infection and inflammation in the bronchii. This condition can result in permanent fibrosis and the dilation of the bronchii. Patients with bronchiectasis will present with elevated bronchovascular marks and parallel lines on the outside of the bronchii. A high-resolution CT scan will often indicate dilated airways and large bulbous cysts at the ends of the bronchii. The diagnosis of bronchiectasis needs to rule out bronchial cysts, eosinophilia, streptococcal pneumonia, cystic fibrosis, and tuberculosis, among other things. Antibiotics can be used to treat any bacterial infections, while severe cases may require lobectomy or lung transplantation. The chest should be drained as necessary.

Hypoxemia

Hypoxemia is a form of acute respiratory failure that can be caused by a number of different things: diminished ventilation, a right-to-left shunt, diffusion impairment, and ventilation perfusion. Patients suffering from hypoxemia are likely to have diminished levels of hyperbaric oxygen saturation, and may also present with altered mental state and pleuritic chest pain. Hypoxemia can be diagnosed after pulse oximetry indicates decrease saturation of hyperbaric oxygen and an arterial blood gas measure indicates an elevated alveolar-arterial gradient. The treatment of hypoxemia depends on the etiology of the case; patients who are already on a ventilator can have their positive end-expiratory pressure increased, and hypercapnic patients can benefit from increased minute ventilation.

Pulmonary thromboembolism

<u>Introduction and symptoms</u> -- A pulmonary thromboembolism is the sudden blockage of one of the pulmonary arteries or its branches; this occlusion may be caused by a blood clot or by some foreign material. Pulmonary thromboembolism usually manifests with Virchow's triad, which consists of statis, endothelial injury, and hypercoagulable states. Patients are more likely to suffer from pulmonary thromboembolism when they have recently undergone congestive heart failure, surgery, or a bone fracture, or use an oral contraceptive. Individuals suffering from pulmonary thromboembolism will present with dyspnea, slight fever, and pleuritic chest pain. A pulmonary embolism manifests as loud P2, hypoxia, and hypocarbia with resulting respiratory alkalosis. Venous thrombosis, on the other hand, presents with unilateral swelling and the appearance of cords on the calf muscle.

<u>Diagnosis and treatment</u> -- If a patient is either hospitalized or confined to bed but displays tachycardia and dyspnea despite a normal chest X ray, this suggests pulmonary embolism. The diagnosis of this condition can be confirmed by a measure of arterial blood gas that indicates respiratory alkalosis, and an ECG that displays sinus tachycardia. The angiogram is the most accurate means of diagnosing this condition, but because it is so invasive it is not usually used. The clot that caused the pulmonary embolism can often be spotted with a venous ultrasound of the lower extremities. Patients suffering from pulmonary thromboembolism should be given heparin, thrombolysis (if there is right heart failure), inferior vena cava filter, and warfarin (in cases where long-term anticoagulation is needed).

Pulmonary hypertension

Pulmonary hypertension can cause permanent damage to the lungs. It is typically caused by diseases of the heart, disorders of the lung parenchyma, or disorders of the pulmonary vessels. A patient suffering from pulmonary hypertension will present with fatigue, dyspnea or syncope on exertion, and edema. It is quite common for patients with pulmonary hypertension to have a history of sickle cell anemia, COPD, emphysema, and pulmonary emboli. The positive diagnosis of pulmonary hypertension can be made after a chest X ray confirms that the central pulmonary arteries have become enlarged and an electrocardiogram indicates right ventricular hypertrophy. Patients suffering from pulmonary hypertension can be given supplemental oxygen diuretics, digoxin, or vasodilators, depending on the etiology of the condition.

Obstructive sleep apnea

Obstructive sleep apnea is characterized by short interruptions of breathing that are caused by some physical obstruction to the airflow. Individuals are more likely to suffer from OSA if they are male, obese, and require sedatives in order to sleep. Patients suffering from obstructive sleep apnea will often present with daytime sleepiness, and their bed partners will report loud snoring. Patients should score normally on pulmonary function tests as long as they are awake. A positive diagnosis of OSA can be made after polysomnography (sleep test) indicates the patient has been aroused from sleep a number of times during the night, and is suffering from some degree of oxygen desaturation while sleeping. The treatment for OSA may entail helping the patient to lose weight, avoid sedatives and alcohol before bed; in extreme cases, tonsillar hypertrophy will need to be corrected with surgery.

Lung cancer

Introduction -- Lung cancer is a malignant tumor of the lung. Lung cancer kills more men and women than does any other kind of cancer. Individuals are more likely to develop lung cancer if they regularly smoke tobacco or if they have been exposed to radon or asbestos. Small cell lung cancer is especially associated with cigarette smoking; it typically has a central location and metastasizes to other areas of the body. Non-small cell lung cancer is less prone to metastasizing, and can be either adenocarcinoma or bronchoalveolar carcinoma. Adenocarcinoma is the most prevalent form of lung cancer. The other types of lung cancer are squamous cell carcinoma and neuroendocrine carcinomas, the latter of which has an especially poor prognosis.

Diagnosis and treatment -- The cells of small-cell lung cancer appear as tiny oats when looked at under a microscope. This kind of cancer cannot be surgically resected; instead, the patient should be given radiation or chemotherapy. Unfortunately, this form of cancer always returns, and is usually not diagnosed at all until it has begun to metastasize. Patients with small-cell cancer typically have a smaller chance of survival than do those with large-cell cancer, which can be surgically resected if it is diagnosed early. This procedure can be traumatic for the patient, so it is important that he or she is in good physical condition before it is performed. In most cases, and depending on the particular type of cancer that is present, the surgery should be accompanied by chemotherapy and radiation.

Lung cancer often presents with hemoptysis, weight loss, irregular breathing, chest pain, and cough. Some patients will present with Horner's syndrome, in which one eyeball is sunken as its lid droops, and the patient does not sweat. Others may have one of the parenoplastic syndromes. The diagnosis of lung cancer can be made after a chest X ray or CT scan reveals a cancerous mass in the lung. In order to confirm the diagnosis, it may be helpful to perform a fine-needle aspiration or bronchoscopy, in which the doctor can examine the breathing passages with the use of a lighted tube. In some cases, a doctor may want to perform a thoroscopic biopsy, which may become a full-blown thoracotomy if the tumor is determined to be malignant.

Lung nodules

Lung nodules are small collections of tissue that form on the internal surface of the lungs. They are often asymptomatic, though some patients will present with dyspnea, shortness of breath, and a recurring cough. In order to make a diagnosis of lung nodules, a doctor should first perform a series of chest X rays in order to determine the size and location of the nodules. A chest CT scan can be used to assess the degree to which the nodules have infiltrated the lung surface. If the patient is older than 45 and has uncalcified lesions larger than 2 cm, then the lesions are likely cancerous. If the patient is younger than 35 and has smaller lesions with smooth borders, then the lesions are likely benign. If the lesion is suspected to be carcinoma, then a surgical resection should be performed.

Pneumothorax

Introduction -- The condition called pneumothorax refers to a collection of free air outside of the lungs in the chest cavity. This condition can ultimately lead to collapse of the lungs. There are three basic kinds of pneumothorax. First degree (spontaneous) pneumothorax is caused by the rupture of subpleual apical blisters (blebs). Second degree pneumothorax is caused tuberculosis, trauma, chronic obstructive pulmonary disease or by some other iatrogenic factor (in other words, by some error in medical treatment). The third and last subtype of pneumothorax is called tension pneumothorax; in this condition, some hole in the chest or lung wall admits air into the pleural cavity. This can be the result of trauma, infection, and the positive-pressure ventilation systems used to treat disorder like sleep apnea. Tension pneumothorax is extremely deadly.

Symptoms, diagnosis, and treatment -- Patients suffering from pneumothorax will often present with one-sided pleuritic chest pain and dyspnea. A closer physical examination will often reveal tachypnea, decreased breathing noises, hyperresonance, and diminished tactile fremitus. If a patient is having a hard time breathing and registers diminished oxygen saturation and tracheal deviation, then the doctor should immediately suspect pneumothorax. If there is time to make a positive diagnosis, the doctor can perform a chest X ray, which will likely show a visceral pleural line and/or movement of the lungs away from the wall of the chest. Minor pneumothoraces can resolve by themselves, but some patients may benefit from oxygen therapy. Other, more serious cases may require the placement of a chest tube, and tension pneumothorax will necessitate needle decompression and chest tube placement.

Nutritional and Digestive Disorders

Acute cholecystitis

Acute cholecystitis is a prolonged obstruction of the cystic duct, a condition typically caused by an impacted stone. This condition can create severe distension, inflammation, and even gangrene of the gallbladder. If a chronically debilitated individual develops the condition without cholelithiasis, this is known as acalculous cholecystitis. Patients with acute cholecystitis will present with nausea, low-grade fever, vomiting, and intense pain in the right upper quadrant. An examination may reveal Murphy's sign, a phenomenon in which there is inspiratory arrest during deep palpation of the right upper quadrant. A positive diagnosis of acute cholecystitis can be made after CBC, amylase, lipase, and LFT panel have been obtained, and an ultrasound indicates stones, bile sludge, pericholecystic fluid, and a thickened gallbladder wall.

If an ultrasound does not rule conclusively on the existence of acute cholecystitis, a hepato-iminodiacetetic acid scan may be administered; if the HIDA scan does not show the gallbladder, then acute cholecystitis is suggested. Patients who are diagnosed with acute cholecystitis should be immediately hospitalized and given intravenous antibiotics, fluids, and electrolytes. An early cholecystectomy should be performed within three days, as should a preoperative ECRP or an intraoperative cholangiogram for the purpose of ruling out common bile duct stones. If the patient has another significant medical problem that precludes surgery, then he or she should be monitored for four to six weeks before surgery to see if the problem resolves spontaneously. Common complications of acute cholecystitis are gangrene, emphysema, perforation, gallstone ileus, fistulization, sepsis, and abscess formation.

Cholelithoasis and biliary colic

The condition known as colic is caused by transient cystic duct blockage created by impacted stones. Doctors often remember the risk factors of colic as the 4 Fs: female, fat, forty, and fertile. Some of the other risk factors of the disorder are oral contraceptive use, rapid weight loss, and a positive family history. Patients with colic will present with abdominal pain after eating that begins in the right upper quadrant and radiates to the right subscapular area or epigastrium. The majority of patients, however, will have asymptomatic gallstones. A positive diagnosis can be made after a right upper quadrant ultrasound indicates gallstones (this procedure, however, is only 85-90% sensitive). Treatment may include cholecystectomy if this is chosen by the patient. Those who seek to avoid surgery should avoid fatty foods.

Choledocholithiasis

Choledocholithiasis is a common condition in which the patient develops gallstones in the common bile duct. The degree and duration of obstruction, as well as the extent of bacterial infection, will determine the level of symptoms. Patients suffering from choledocholithiasis may not have any symptoms at all, but some will present with biliary pain, jaundice, episodic colic , fever, and pancreatitis. A positive diagnosis of the condition can be made after elevated alkaline phosphatase and total bilirubin are indicated. Treatment for choledocholithiasis typically includes endoscopic retrograde cholangiopancreatography accompanied by sphincterectomy. After this, the patient may receive cholecystectomy if he or she so chooses.

Acute cholangitis

Acute cholangitis is an acute bacterial infection of the biliary tree that usually occurs as a result of obstruction that is either caused by gallstones or first degree sclerosing cholangitis. Some of the more commonly identified pathogens associated with the condition are gram-negative enterics, as for instance E. Coli. Individuals may be at a heightened risk of developing acute cholangitis if they have bile duct stricture, ampullary carcinoma, and pancreatic pseudocyst. Patients will typically present with what is known as Charcot's triad: pain in the right upper quadrant, jaundice, and fever or chills. Patients with acute suppurative cholangitis accompanied by sepsis may present what is known as Renolds' pentad: that is, Charcot's triad plus shock and altered mental status.

In order to make a positive diagnosis of acute cholangitis, one should examine the patient for leukocytosis, elevated biluribuin, and elevated alkaline phosphatase. In order to exclude the possibility of sepsis, a blood culture should be obtained. Although most of the time the diagnosis will be based on clinical impression, an ultrasound or a CT may be helpful. Some patients may benefit from an endoscopic retrograde cholangiopancreatography. Treatment for acute cholangitis usually includes admission to the intesnive care unit for the purpose of monitoring, hydration, blood pressure support, and broad-spectrum antibiotic treatment. The crucial step in treating patients with acute cholangitis is to administer emergent bile duct decompression by means of open decompression, ECRP sphincterectomy, and percutaneous transhepatic drainage.

Diarrhea

An individual is suffering from diarrhea when he or she has a change in stool consistency and is producing more than 200 grams of stool every day. Risk factors for diarrhea include viral or bacterial gastro-intestinal infection, systemic infection, contact with another sick person, immunosuppression, recent travel, or recent use of antibiotics. Diarrhea may be classified as either acute, chronic, or pediatric. Acute diarrhea is infectious and self-limited, and usually has less than three weeks of symptoms. Chronic diarrhea, on the other hand, has an insidious onset with more than 6 weeks of symptoms, and is typically caused by disrupted secretion, altered motility, celiac sprue, bacterial overgrowth, irritable bowel disorder, or lactose intolerance. Pediatric diarrhea is most often due to rotavirus infection.

A positive diagnosis of diarrhea can be made based on clinical impression for the most part, though the diagnosis of chronic diarrhea may require that a stool sample be sent for fecal leukocytes, bacterial culture, the C. difficile toxin, and ova and parasites. Patients with bloody diarrhea may require sigmoidoscopy. If a patient is diagnosed with acute diarrhea and bacterial infection is not suspected, then the patient should be given antidiarrheals and fluid replacement with electrolytes. If there is an indication of systemic infection, on the other hand, then the patient should be given antibiotics and should be cautioned away from antimotility agents. The underlying cause of chronic diarrhea should be treated with loperamide, opioids, octreotide, or cholestyramine.

Infectious diarrhea

Caused by salmonella or shigella -- A person may develop diarrhea from salmonella if he or she ingests contaminated poultry or eggs. This infection generally lasts between two and five days and is accompanied by prodromal headache, fever, myalgia, and abdominal pain. Once the diagnosis has been made, treatment should make sure that sepsis does not develop, as patients may become bacteremic. Those patients who do become bacteremic or are considered to be at risk of doing so should be given oral quinolone or TMP-SMX. Another form of infectious diarrhea is caused by shigella. This variety of infection is extremely contagious and is transmitted by the fecal-oral route. The danger of shigella-caused diarrhea is that it may lead to severe dehydration or to febrile seizures in very young patients. This infection should be treated with TMP-SMX in order to diminish the risk of interpersonal contamination.

Caused by entamoeba histolytica and E. Coli -- Individuals may develop diarrhea after ingesting food or water that is contaminated with the bacteria entamoeba histolytica. This form of diarrhea is especially common among people who have recently traveled to developing countries. Patients with this form of diarrhea are likely to present with severe abdominal pain and fever. Because steroids can lead to a fatal perforation, patients should always be treated with metronidazole. Another severe form of diarrhea is caused by the E. Coli bacteria. This bacteria is ingested in food, and is most dangerous to children and the elderly. The diarrhea stemming from E. Coli typically lasts between five and ten days, and may be accompanied by low-grade fever, vomiting, and severe abdominal pain. In order to give a positive diagnosis, both gastro-intestinal bleeding and ischemic colitis should be excluded. Patients with this form of diarrhea should not be given antibiotics.

Caused by campylobacter and clostridium difficile -- Campylobacter is the most common cause of infectious diarrhea. It is transmitted through the ingestion of contaminated food or water, and is more likely to affect children and young adults. The diarrhea caused by campylobacter typically lasts between a week and twelve days. In order diagnose this kind of diarrhea, irritable bowel disorder and appendicitis should be ruled out. Erythromicin is the most common treatment for diarrhea caused by campylobacter. Diarrhea may also be caused by clostridium difficile after antibiotic treatment. Patients with this form of diarrhea are likely to present with fever, abdominal pain, and systemic toxicity. This condition is most commonly located in the large bowel. Patients may be given oral metronidazole or oral vancomycin.

Irritable bowel syndrome

Irritable bowel syndrome is an idiopathic functional disorder in which the individual has severe abdominal pain and changes in bowel habits. These problems will be magnified by stress and diminished by bowel movements. Most of the time, an individual suffering from

IBS will also have a psychiatric disorder like depression or anxiety. Typically, patients will present with abdominal pain and distension, and stools with mucus. A positive diagnosis of IBS can be made after CBC, TSH, electrolytes, stool cultures, abdominal films, and barium contrast studies rule out other gastrointestinal disorders. Treatment is tripartite: evaluation and assistance with the underlying psychological problems; fiber supplements and a general improvement in diet; and TCAs, antidiarrheals, antispasmodics, and tegaserod.

Small bowel obstruction

Introduction -- A small bowel obstruction (a blocked passage of bowel contents) can lead to an excess of fluid and gas as well as electrolyte imbalances. This can be extremely painful. Obstruction may be partial or complete, and it is possible for the bowel to become entirely strangled. SBO may be caused by the following: adhesions from a prior abdominal surgery; hernias; neoplasms; intussusception; gallstone ileus, stricture due to irritable bowel syndrome, volvulus, or cystic fibrosis. Patients with this disorder typically present with cramping abdominal pain that occurs in a rising and falling pattern that lasts five or ten minutes. This pain is often followed by vomiting; if the obstruction is proximal the emesis will be bilious, but if it is distal the emesis will be feculent. Individuals with partial obstruction will have flatus but no stool, while individuals with complete obstruction will have obstipation.

Symptoms -- An abdominal exam of an individual with a small bowel obstruction will typically reveal distention, tenderness, prior surgical scars, or hernias. The bowel sounds most commonly heard in patients with SBO are high-pitched tinkles and peristaltic rushes. If the patient develops fever, hypotension, rebound tenderness, or tachycardia then immediate surgery is necessary. A positive diagnosis of SBO can be made if a complete blood count demonstrates leukocytosis, which will be the case if there is strangulation of the bowel. Also, chemistry may indicate dehydration and metabolic alkalosis caused by frequent vomiting, while lactic acidosis suggests necrotic bowel and indicates that immediate surgery is required.

Diagnosis and treatment -- A positive diagnosis of small bowel obstruction can be made when abdominal films indicate a step-ladder pattern of dilated small-bowel loops, air fluid levels, and a smaller than normal amount of gas in the colon. Gallstone ileus is suggested by radiopaque material at the cecum. A partial obstruction in the small bowel may only require supportive care, such as nasogastric suction, intravenous hydration, correction of electrolyte abnormalities, and Foley catheterization to monitor fluid status. If the patient has a complete obstruction, vascular compromise, or symptoms lasting more than three days, then surgery should be performed. Sometimes an exploratory laparotomy will be performed along with a lysis of adhesions, a resection of a necrotic bowel, and evaluation for stricture, irritable bowel disorder, and hernias.

Ileus

Symptoms -- Ileus is the loss of peristaltis without there being a structural obstruction. Individuals are at greater risk of ileus when they have had recent surgery or gastrointestinal procedures, severe medical illness, immobility, hypokalemia, hypothyroidism, diabetes mellitus, and medications like anticholinergics and opioids that slow down gastrointestinal motility. Patients with ileus present with abdominal discomfort, nausea, vomiting, and an absence of flatulence or bowel movements. There may also be abdominal tenderness, an absence of peritoneal sounds, and a decrease in or absence of bowel sounds. Elderly patients should receive a rectal examination in order to rule out fecal impaction.

Diagnosis and treatment -- A positive diagnosis of ileus can be made after diffusely distended loops of the small and large bowel are visible on a supine abdominal X ray and air-fluid levels can be seen on an upright view. In order to exclude the possibility of partial obstruction, a Gastrogafin study may be performed. In order to exclude the possibility of neoplasms, it may be necessary to perform a CT. As for treatment, the patient should decrease or terminate the use of any medications that decrease motility, as for instance narcotics. Also, the patient should temporarily diminish or discontinue oral feeding. In some cases, it may be helpful to administer nasogastric suction or parenteral feeds. Also, electrolytes should be repleted if this is indicated.

Malabsorption

Malabsorption is a condition in which the patient cannot absorb nutrients; this problem is caused by some underlying disorder like celiac disease, Whipple's disease, short bowel syndrome, pancreatic insufficiency, lactose intolerance, and infection. The patient may have diminished absorption of protein, fat, carbohydrates, and the smaller vitamins and minerals. Patients suffering from malabsorption will present with frequent loose stools and/or pale, smelly, bulky stools. Patients may also have flatus, bloating, weight loss, fatigue, and nutritional deficiencies. Treatment for malabsorption depends on the etiology. Severe cases may benefit from total parenteral nutrition, immunosuppressants, and anti-inflammatory medication.

Diverticular disease

Introduction and symptoms -- Diverticular disease is manifested in outpouchings of the mucosa and submucosa that herniated through the colonic muscle layers in regions where there is high intraluminal pressure. Diverticular disease is most commonly manifested in the sigmoid colon. For patients more than 40 years old, diverticulosis is the most common cause of acute gastro-intestinal bleeding. The risk factors for diverticular disease include a low-fiber and high-fat diet, advanced age, and connective tissue disorders like Marfan's and Ehlers-Danlos syndromes. Diverticulitis is specifically caused by an inflammation and possible perforation of a diverticulum. Patients with diverticular disease will often present with no symptoms, though there may be constipation, abdominal pain in the lower left quadrant, and abnormal bowel habits.

Diagnosis and treatment -- Patients with diverticulitis will present with an acute, mild-to-severe pain in the lower left quadrant accompanied by fever, nausea, and vomiting. A positive diagnosis of diverticular disease can be made after a complete blood count indicates leukocytosis, and the condition is corroborated by abdominal X ray, colonoscopy, or barium enema. In severe cases, a CT may indicate abscess or free air. Patients with uncomplicated diverticular disease should be monitored and placed on a high fiber diet. In cases of diverticular bleeding, the patient should be given fluids and transfusions as necessary until the bleeding stops of its own accord. In the rare instances where this does not occur, an angiography with embolization or surgery will be required. Diverticulitis should be treated with bowel rest, nasogastric tube placement, and broad-spectrum antibiotics. If there is perforation, an immediate surgical resection should be performed.

Carcinoid syndrome

Carcinoid syndrome is caused by lever metastasis of serotonin and substance P from carcinoid tumors. These usually arise out of the appendix or the ileum. Patients with carcinoid syndrome will likely present with cutaneous flushing, wheezing, diarrhea, and cardiac valvular lesions. Patients are most likely to suffer from adverse symptoms after eating, exertion, or excitement. A positive diagnosis of carcinoid syndrome can be made after a urine test indicates high levels of the serotonin metabolite 5-HIAA. A chest and/or abdominal CT scan can be used to determine the precise location of the tumor. Treatment for carcinoid syndrome typically entails a reduction of the tumor mass and octeotride for symptoms.

Large bowel obstruction

Introduction and symptoms -- A large bowel obstruction may be caused by colon cancer, diverticulitis, volvulus, fecal impaction, and benign tumors. A patient suffering from a large bowel obstruction will often present with constipation/obstipation, cramping abdominal pain, and nausea or vomiting. A physical examination will reveal distension, tympany, and tenderness, as well as high-pitched bowel noises. The patient should be examined for peritoneal irritation or mass; if fever or shock symptoms are present, then the patient may be experiencing perforation/peritonitis or ischemia/strangulation. An examining doctor should always assume that the cause of the large bowel obstruction is colon cancer until another cause is determined.

Diagnosis and treatment -- A positive diagnosis of large bowel obstruction can be made after a complete blood count, electrolytes, lactic acid, abdominal X ray, CT scan, water contrast enema, and sigmoidoscopy or colonoscopy have been performed. The examining doctor should be sure to differentiate large bowel obstruction from small bowel obstruction, paralytic ileus, appendicitis, and irritable bowel disorder. The patient should be immediately hospitalized, and the obstruction should be treated with a Gastrografin enema, colonoscopy, or a rectal tube. In most cases, surgery will be required. If the patient has a gangrenous colon, then a partial colectomy with a diverting colostomy needs to be performed. Also, it is important that the underlying cause of the obstruction be treated.

Colon and rectal cancer

Introduction and symptoms -- Individuals are more likely to develop colon or rectal cancer as they increase in age. There are also a number of hereditary syndromes that increase the likelihood of colorectal cancer: familial adenomatous polyposis, Gardner's disease, and hereditary nonpolyposis colorectal cancer. Individuals with irritable bowel disorder are more likely to develop colorectal cancer, especially is they have ulcerative colitis. Finally, individuals are at a greater risk of colorectal cancer if they have a high-fat, low-fiber diet. In order to screen for colorectal cancer, individuals older than 50 should receive an annual digital rectal examination and stool guaiac. More than half of the lesions indicative of colorectal cancer can be identified by a sigmoidoscopy, so these should be performed every 3 to 5 years. If a patient has a family history of colorectal cancer, he or she should receive a colonoscopy every 10 years after the age of 40.

Unless colorectal cancer is identified in screening, it usually is discovered after a long period of silent growth. The most common presenting complaint is abdominal pain. Lesions may be either right- or left-sided or rectal. Right-sided lesions are often bulky, ulcerating masses that can lead to anemia from chronic occult blood loss. Patients with right-sided lesions may complain of weight loss, anorexia, diarrhea, weakness, or vague abdominal pain. Left-sided lesions, on the other hand, are usually obstructing masses that resemble an apple core. Patients with left-sided lesions will complain of a change in bowel habits and/or blood-streaked stools. Patients suffering from rectal lesions often will present with bright red blood in the rectum, possible accompanied by tenesmus and/or rectal pain. Rectal lesions may exist at the same time as hemorrhoids, which can often confuse a diagnosis.

Diagnosis -- In order to diagnose colorectal cancer, a doctor should first obtain a complete blood count and a stool occult blood. A sigmoidoscopy should be performed in order to examine rectal bleeding and any left-sided lesions. A colonoscopy can be performed in order to rule out synchronous right-sided lesions. Sometimes a colonoscopy will be incomplete, in which case an air-contrast barium enema can be used to exclude the possibility of additional lesions. An endoscopic ultrasound may be used to determine the degree of invasion of rectal cancer. Colon cancer is staged according to Dukes' criteria using a whole-body CT/MRI. It is also a good idea to administer a chest X-ray, abdominal CT, and liver function test to provide a metastatic workup.

Treatment -- Treatment for colorectal cancer should begin with a preoperative bowel prep, which entails mechanical stool evacuation. Colonic lesions should be treated with surgical resection of the lesions, as well as resection of the lymphatic drainage and mesentery at the origin of the arterial blood supply. The proper technique for treating abdominal lesions depends on the proximity of the lesion to the anal verge, which is the meeting of the anal canal and anal skin. In the case of low-lying lesions that are less than 10 cm from the anal canal, an abdominoperineal resection should be performed in which the rectum and anus are resected and a permanent colostomy is established. In the case of proximal lesions more than 10 cm from the anal verge, a low anterior resection should be performed, meaning that a first degree anastomosis between the colon and the rectum should be created. If the patient has small, well-differentiated tumors in the lower third of his or her rectum, then a wide local excision should be made. If colon cancer exists along with positive nodes, adjuvant chemotherapy is recommended.

Dysphagea/odynophagia

Dysphagea is difficulty in swallowing, and odynophagea is a complete inability to swallow. These conditions are caused by abnormalities of the oropharynx or esophagus. Causes may include achalasia, peptic stricture, esophageal webs or rings, carcinoma, scleroderma, spastic motility disorders, medications, and radiation injury. Oropharyngeal dysphagia is usually more of a problem with liquids than solids, while esophageal dysphagia is just the opposite. A positive diagnosis of oropharyngeal dysphagia can be made after a cine-esophagram, while a positive diagnosis of esophageal dysphagia requires a barium swallow followed by endoscopy, manometry, and/or pH monitoring. Odynphagia can be diagnosed with an upper endoscopy. The treatment for these conditions depends on the etiology.

Gastroesophageal reflux disease

Introduction and symptoms -- Gastroesophageal reflux disease (GERD) is a persistent reflux of the gastric contents into the esophagus. This condition is usually a result of transient lower esophageal sphincter relaxation. Individuals are at a greater risk of GERD when they have increased intra-abdominal pressure due to obesity or pregnancy, or when they have scleroderma, alcoholism, or consume nicotine, caffeine, chocolate or fatty foods. Patients with this condition will typically present with heart burn half an hour to ninety minutes after a meal. Also, patients may complain of a sour taste in their mouth, laryngitis, wheezing, or dysphagia. An examination will be normal unless some systemic disease is also present.

Diagnosis and treatment -- A positive diagnosis of GERD can be based on clinical impression and history, though it may be useful to perform an abdominal X ray, chest X ray, barium swallow, esophageal manometry, and 24-hour pH monitoring. If the patient has had symptoms for a long period, it may be necessary to perform an esophagogastroduodenoscopy in order to exclude the possibility of Barrett's esophagus and adenocarcinoma. Treatment for this condition should include lifestyle changes like weight loss and the avoidance of foods that tend to decrease lower esophageal sphincter tone. Patients that have intermittent GERD should be given antacids, while patients with more chronic conditions should be given H2 receptor antagonists and PPIs.

Esophageal cancer

The two most common types of esophageal cancer are squamous cell carcinoma and adenocarcinoma. Adenocarcinoma is often accompanied by Barrett's esophagus, in which there is columnar metaplasia of the distal esophagus after chronic gastroesophageal reflux disease. Individuals are at a greater risk of esophageal cancer if they smoke or abuse alcohol. Patients will normally present with progressive dysphagia, weight loss, gastroesophageal reflux disease, gastrointestinal bleeding, and vomiting. A positive diagnosis can be made after a barium study indicates a narrowing of the esophagus with an irregular border extending into the lumen. An EGD or biopsy can be used to confirm the result. Chemoradiation therapy and surgical resection are both often used for treatment, though neither is especially effective.

Hiatal hernia

A hiatal hernia is a herniation of some part of the stomach up into the chest through a diaphragmatic opening. By far the most common kind of hiatal hernia is a sliding hiatal hernia, in which the gastroesophageal junction and part of the stomach are moved above the diaphragm. Much less common is the paraesophageal hiatal hernia, in which the junction of the stomach and esophagus remains below the diaphragm, but a nearby portion of the fundus is displaced into the mediastinum. Hiatal hernias may be asymptomatic, and are frequently discovered on a chest X ray by accident. Treatment for a sliding hernia entails changes in lifestyle to reduce the symptoms of GERD; paraesophageal hernias can be treated with surgical gastropexy in order to prevent gastric volvulus.

Gastritis

Introduction and symptoms -- Gastritis is quite simply an inflammation of the stomach lining. Acute gastritis is characterized by superficial lesions that develop quickly and are often caused by NSAIDs, alcohol, or stress from a severe injury. There are two types of chronic gastritis. Type A gastritis is very rare and is usually due to autoantibodies to parietal cells. Type A gastritis occurs in the fundus and is linked to other autoimmune disorders like pernicious anemia and thyroiditis. Also, individuals with Type A gastritis have an elevated risk of adenocarcinoma. Type B chronic gastritis is much more common and is usually caused by NSAID use or H. pylori infection. Type B gastritis occurs in the antrum, and though it is often asymptomatic, it is also thought to increase the risk of peptic ulcer disease and gastric cancer.

Diagnosis and treatment -- Individuals suffering from gastritis may display no symptoms at all, though they may also complain of indigestion, nausea, hematemesis, melena, or vomiting. In order to make a positive diagnosis of gastritis, a doctor may need to get a visual representation of the gastric lining, in which case he or she will benefit from an upper endoscopy. The following tests can be used to determine whether a patient has an H. pylori infection: urease breath test, serum IgG antibody, urine H. pylori stool antigen, or endoscopic biopsy. As for treatment, patients should immediately decrease their consumption of the irritating substances. Many will benefit from antacids, sucralfate, H2 blockers, and PPIs. Patients who are considered to be at risk of a stress ulcer should receive prophylactic H2 blockers.

Peptic ulcer disease

Introduction and symptoms -- Peptic ulcer disease is any damage to the duodenal or gastric mucosa that is caused by either damaged mucosal defenses or elevated acid in the gastric system. The vast majority of ulcers in both the duodenal and gastric systems are caused by H. pylori. Individuals are also considered to be at a greater risk of PUD if they smoke, drink heavily, or consume non-steroidal anti-inflammatory drugs or corticosteroids. It is more likely that a male rather than a female will be afflicted by peptic ulcers. Patients suffering from PUD typically present with either chronic or regular burning epigastric pain that is much better after a meal. The pain will typically return two or three hours after the meal. Occasionally, patients will present with nausea, hematemesis, or bloody stool.

Diagnosis -- Patients suffering from peptic ulcer disease may show epigastric tenderness or a positive stool guiac during examination. If the patient presents with a firm abdomen, guarding, or any other sign of peritoneal irritation, he or she may have an acute perforation. In order to make a positive diagnosis of PUD, an abdominal X ray should be performed so that perforation can be ruled out; similarly, a complete blood count should be taken to assess the general level of gastro-intestinal bleeding. The diagnosis of PUD can be confirmed by an upper endoscopy with biopsy; this procedure can also be used to exclude a diagnosis of active bleeding or gastric adenocarcinoma. The following tests can be used to test for H. pylori: urease breath test, serum IgG, stool H. pylori antigen, or endoscopic biopsy.

Treatment -- In cases of acute peptic ulcer disease, the doctor's first move is to exclude the possibility of active bleeding with a nasogastric lavage, rectal exam with stool guaiac, and serial hematocrit. If it becomes evident that perforation has occurred, then emergent surgery should be performed. The pharmacological treatment for PUD entails decreasing acid production, eliminating any H. pylori infection, and protecting the mucosa. Mild cases of PUD can be treated with antacids, while cases of H. pylori infection should be given triple therapy: amoxicillin, clarithromycin, and omeprazole. If a patient suffers from symptomatic gastric ulcers for more than two months, then he or she should have either an endoscopy or an upper gastrointestinal series with barium in order to exclude the possibility of adenocarcinoma. There are four main complications of PUD: hemorrhage, obstruction, perforation, and intractable pain.

Gastric cancer

One of the most common causes of death is gastric cancer. There are two morphological types of these malignant tumors, which are generally adenocarcinomas. The diffuse type are usually poorly differentiated, and do not have anything to do with H. pylori infection or chronic gastritis. The intestinal type of tumor is believed to develop because of intestinal metaplasia of gastric mucosal cells. Individuals are at a greater risk of intestinal tumors when they have a diet high in nitrites and salt and low in fresh vegetables. Patients will typically present with abdominal pain, early satiety, and weight loss. A positive diagnosis of gastric cancer can be made after endoscopic examination. The condition is typically asymptomatic until it is quite advanced. Treatment is only successful when the cancer is detected and removed early.

Upper GI bleeding

Individuals may develop upper gastrointestinal bleeding as a result of gastritis, peptic ulcer disease, a Mallory-Weiss tear, esophageal varices, vascular abnormalities, neoplasm, or esophagitis. Patients with this condition will typically present with hematemesis and a depleted volume status (causing, for example, tachycardia, light-headedness, or hypotension). The positive diagnosis of upper GI bleeding can be made after a nasogastric tube and lavage have been inserted; it may be appropriate to perform an endoscopy if the patient is stable.

Treatment should aim first to stabilize the patient, and then to protect the airway, possibly with intubation. More generally, treatment will be aimed at resolving the underlying causes of the bleeding.

Lower GI bleeding

Individuals may develop lower gastrointestinal bleeding as a result of diverticulosis, atrioventricular malformations, neoplasm, irritable bowel disorder, anorectal disease, or mesenteric ischemia. Patients are likely to present with hematochezia greater than melena, although this is not always the case. A positive diagnosis of lower GI bleeding can be made after upper GI bleeding has been ruled out by a nasogastric lavage and intubation. If the patient is stable, a colonoscopy may be helpful in making the diagnosis. The initial treatment for lower GI bleeding is aimed at stabilizing the patient with intravenous fluids and blood; afterwards, treatment should aim at managing the underlying cause of the bleeding.

Zollinger-Ellison syndrome

Individuals suffering from Zollinger-Ellison syndrome develop gastrin-producing tumors in the pancreas and/or the duodenum that result in an oversecretion of gastrin. When there is an excessive level of gastrin, there are also high levels of gastric acid, and so the patient will develop persistent and painful ulcers in the stomach and duodenum. Patients will typically present with a burning abdominal pain that is unresponsive to treatment; other common symptoms include diarrhea, nausea, vomiting, fatigue, weakness, weight loss, and gastro-intestinal bleeding. In order to make a positive diagnosis of Zollinger-Ellison syndrome, a doctor must measure the serum gastrin level and perform an endoscopic examination of the gastric mucosa. Treatment for this condition entails diminishing acid production, often with the aid of a PPI.

Inguinal hernias

Inguinal hernias are abnormal protrusions of the contents of the abdominal cavity into the inguinal region. These contents protrude through a weakness or injury to the abdominal wall. An indirect hernia extends through the internal and external inguinal rings and, in males, may eventually protrude into the scrotum. Indirect hernias are more common in both males and females, and are blamed on a congenital patent processus vaginalis. Direct hernias involve when the abdominal contents protrude through Hesselbach's triangle. In this type of hernia, the sac contents do not traverse the internal inguinal ring, but rather protrude directly through the abdominal wall and into the aponeurosis of the external oblique muscle. This condition is usually due to an acquired defect in the transversalis fascia. Open or laparoscopic surgery is usually required, as there is always a risk of incarceration and strangulation.

Ulcerative colitis

Introduction and symptoms -- Ulcerative colitis affects the rectum and typically extends proximally in a continuous manner. The inflammation and ulceration associated with this condition are typically limited to the mucosa and the submucosa. Patients with this condition will typically present with bloody diarrhea, tenesmus, urgency, and lower abdominal cramps. A physical examination will often indicate orthostatic hypotension, tachycardia, abdominal tenderness, frank blood on rectal exam, and extraintestinal manifestations. These extraintestinal manifestations may include aphthous stomatitis, arthritis, first degree sclerosing cholangitis, toxic megacolon, erythema nodosum, and pyoderma gangrenosum.

Diagnosis and treatment -- Ulcerative colitis can be diagnosed after a complete blood count, abdominal X ray, stool cultures, ova and parasite study, and stool assay have been used to rule out C. difficile. A colonoscopy may show diffuse and continuous rectal involvement, friability, edema, and sometimes pseudopolyps. A positive diagnosis of ulcerative colitis can be made after a biopsy. Treatment for the condition is the administration of sulfasalazine or 5-ASA; refractory disease can be treated with corticsteroids and immunosuppressants. If the patient has toxic megacolon or perisistent/fulminative colitis, then a total colectomy is recommended. Patients who have ulcerative colotis for a long period of time are much more likely to develop ulcerative colitis.

Crohn's disease

Introduction and symptoms -- Crohn's disease is a discontinuous pattern of lesions that can occur anywhere in the gastrointestinal tract, especially the ileolocal region. It is less likely that there will be any lesions in the rectum. Patients with Crohn's disease typically present with abdominal pain, abdominal mass, slight fever, weight loss, and diarrhea. A physical examination will often indicate these symptoms as well as perianal fissures, fistulas, and extra-intestinal manifestations. These extra-intestinal manifestations are similar to the ones suffered by individuals with ulcerative colitis, although there may also be nephrolithiasis and fistulas to the skin, biliary or urinary tract, or between bowel loops.

Diagnosis and treatment -- When Crohn's disease is suspected, the patient should receive the same laboratory examination as if he or she had ulcerative colitis. A colonoscopy may reveal aphthoid, linear, or stellate ulcers, strictures, and cobblestone-like or discontinuous lesions. The definitive diagnosis of Crohn's disease can only be made after a biopsy. Patients who are diagnosed with Crohn's disease should be given sulfasalazine, and if there is no improvement, corticosteroids and immunosuppression. If the patient has endured a perforation, then surgical resection will be necessary. It should be noted that Crohn's disease can recur anywhere in the gastro-intestinal tract. More positively for those with this condition, Crohn's disease is much less likely to lead to a second degree malignancy than is ulcerative colitis.

Hepatitis

Introduction and symptoms -- Hepatitis is an inflammation of the liver. One of the major clinical features of hepatitis is jaundice, which occurs in cases where there is too much bilirubin in the bloodstream. Adults tend to develop jaundice for the following reasons: obstruction of the biliary system, as by an infection, stone, stricture, or tumor; hepatitis; or alcoholic cirrhosis, pancreatic cancer, hemolytic anemia, and congenital disorders of bilurubin metabolism. For adults, jaundice typically means either that the liver is damaged or overloaded, or that the biliary system is unable for some reason to excrete bilurubin. Individuals suffering from hepatitis will typically present with a viral prodrome of nonspecific symptoms like malaise, fever, joint pain, nausea, and vomiting; these symptoms will be succeeded by pain in the right upper quadrant and jaundice.

Diagnosis and treatment -- When an individual with hepatitis is examined, it is quite possible that jaundice, scleretal icterus, tender hepatomegaly, splenomegaly, and lymphadenopathy. Individuals with chronic hepatitis will likely exhibit the symptoms commonly associated with chronic liver disease: jaundice, cirrhosis, and fatigue. Most of the people who have hepatitis C (and at least ten percent of those with hepatitis B) will develop chronic hepatitis. Individuals may be suspected of having hepatitis when they have a normal white blood cell count and very high alanine aminotransferase and aspartate aminotransferase; patients with acute hepatitis will likely also have elevated bilurubin/alkaline phosphatase levels.

Individuals with chronic hepatitis will have an elevated alanine aminotransferase and aspartate aminotransferase for more than 6 months, along with concurrent elevated alkaline phosphatase/bilurubin and hypoalbuminemia. Viral hepatitis can be diagnosed after hepatitis serology or, in severe cases, after a liver biopsy is performed. The treatment of hepatitis depends on the particular etiology of the case. Hepatitis that is caused by severe alcoholism is usually treated with steroids, while hepatitis caused by autoimmune hepatitis is usually treated with immunosuppression featuring steroids and azathioprine. A chronic hepatitis B infection is treated with IFN-alpha, lamiduvine, and adefovir; chronic hepatitis C infection is treated with peginterferon and ribavarin. Patients who are experiencing the final stages of liver failure should be given a liver transplant. Patients with fulminant hepatitic failure require admittance to the intensive care unit and an emergent transplant.

Portal hypertension

Introduction -- Portal hypertension is defined as portal pressure that is 5 mmHg greater than the pressure in the inferior vena cava. The causes of portal hypertension can be presinusoidal, sinusoidal, postsinusoidal, and Budd-Chiari syndrome. Presinusoidal causes include splenic or portal vein thrombosis, schistosomiasis, and granulomatous disease. Sinusoidal causes include cirrhosis and granulomatous disease. Postsinusoidal causes include right heart failure, constrictive pericarditis, and hepatitic vein thrombosis. Portal hypertension can also be caused by Budd-Chiari syndrome, in which there is hepatitic vein thrombosis after hypercoagulability. Patients with this form of portal hypertension have a poor prognosis; they should be given clot lysis, TIPS, or hepatic transplantation.

Diagnosis -- A patient with portal hypertension will typically present with jaundice, ascites, spontaneous bacterial peritonitis, hepatic encephalopathy, gastro-esophageal varices, and renal dysfunction. A closer physical examination often reveals the stigmata associated with portal hypertension. In order to diagnose portal hypertension, a doctor should perform liver function tests, alkaline phosphatase, bilirubin, albumin, and PT/PTT in order to assess hepatic function. In order to determine additional causes like hemochromatosis, Wilson's disease, alpha-antitrypsin deficiency, and Budd-Chiari syndrome, it may be necessary to perform tests like serum ferritin, ceruloplasmin, alpha-antitrypsin, and ultrasound. A patient with portal hypertension will have an elevated indirect heoatic vein wedge pressure.

Treatment -- In order to determine the etiology of ascites in cases of portal hypertension, a doctor should measure the serum ascites albumin gradient, which is found by subtracting the serum albumin from ascites albumin. All of the treatment for portal hypertension is aimed at mitigating the complications. Ascites should be treated with sodium restriction and a program of diuretics, as for instance furosemide and spironolactone. Infectious and neoplastic causes of ascites should be ruled out, and when it is possible the underlying liver disease should be treated. Spontaneous bacterial peritonitis can be treated with intravenous antibiotics, while hepatorenal syndrome may require dialysis. Hepatic encephalopathy can be treated by decreasing the patient's consumption of protein and administering lactulose and/or metronidazole.

Hemochromatosis

Introduction and symptoms -- Hemochromatosis is caused by excessive absorption of iron accompanied by parenchymal hemosiderin accumulation in the liver, pancreas, heart, adrenals, testes, pituitary, and kidneys. Hemochromatosis almost always occurs in men with Northern European ancestry who are fifty years of age or older. It is possible for alcoholics or individuals receiving chronic transfusion therapy to develop second degree hemochromatosis. Patients with hemochromatosis will typically present with abdominal pain, symptoms of diabetes mellitus, hypogonadism, arthropathy of the MCP joints, heart failure, or cirrhosis. A more complete physical examination may reveal bronze skin pigmentation, hepatomegaly, testicular atrophy, pancreatic dysfunction, and cardiac dysfunction.

Treatment and diagnosis -- In order to make a positive diagnosis of hemochromatosis, a doctor should determine whether serum iron levels are elevated, should measure the percent saturation with iron, and should measure ferritin with decrease serum transferrin. The most sensitive and indicative diagnostic test is a fasting transferring saturation of more that 45%. Many patients with hemochromatosis will have glucose intolerance and slightly elevated aspartate aminotransferase and alkaline phosphatase. It may also be necessary in order to make the diagnosis to perform a liver biopsy, hepatic MRI, or hemachromatosis mutation C282Y screen. The treatment for hemochromatosis includes weekly phlebotomy until serum iron levels drop. Maintenance of low serum iron levels can also include deferoxamine. The serious complications of hemochromatosis include cirrhosis and hepatocellular carcinoma.

Hepatocellular carcinoma

Hepatocellular carcinoma is associated with cirrhosis and chronic hepatitis. Patients with hepatocellular carcinoma will often present with right upper quadrant tenderness, abdominal distension, and symptoms commonly associated with liver disease like jaundice, easy bruisability, and coagulopathy. A more complete physical examination will often reveal a nodular cirrhotic liver. A positive diagnosis of hepatocellular carcinoma is made when an ultrasound or CT scan displays a mass, and when the patient is found to have elevated results on a liver function test and extremely high levels of alpha-fetoprotein. In order to be sure, though, a liver biopsy must be performed. If the tumors are caught early in their development, it may be possible to resect or perform an orthotopic liver transplantation. The only practical use of chemotherapy and radiation is to shrink large tumors before surgery.

Wilson's disease

Wilson's disease, also known as hepatolenticular degeneration, is a decreased amount of ceruloplsm and an excessive deposition of copper in the liver and brain. This condition is caused by a deficient copper-transporting protein. Patients with Wilson's disease will typically present with hemolytic anemia, liver abnormalities, and neurological and psychiatric problems like psychosis, mania, anxiety, tremor, and loss of coordination. A more complete physical examination often displays Kayser-Fleischer rings: greenish-brown deposits of copper in Descemet's membrane. Patients may also display jaundice, hepatomegaly, asterixis, chloreiform movements, and rigidity. A positive diagnosis of Wilson's disease can be made after tests indicate decreased serum ceruloplasm , increased urinary copper excretion, and increased hepatic copper. The treatment for this condition includes dietary copper restriction, penicillamine, and oral zinc.

Acute pancreatitis

Introduction and symptoms -- Acute pancreatitis occurs when pancreatic enzymes are leaking into the pancreatic and peripancreatic tissue, often as a result of gallstone disease or alcoholism. Acute pancreatitis typically has a quick onset in which there is severe pain, and is more likely to affect individuals who suffer from gallstones, alcoholism, hypercalcemia, hypertriglyceridemia, trauma, viral infections, post-ECRP, or scorpion bites. A patient suffering from acute pancreatitis will typically present with severe epigastric pain, nausea, vomiting, weakness, fever, and shock; a more comprehensive physical exam may reveal flank discoloration (known as the Grey Turner sign) and periumbilical discoloration (known as Cullen's sign).

Diagnosis and treatment -- A positive diagnosis of acute pancreatitis can be made when lab tests indicate elevated levels of amylase, lipase, and a decreased level of calcium (in severe cases). An ultrasound or CT scan will often indicate an enlarged pancreas with stranding, abscess, hemorrhage, necrosis, or pseudoscyst. The most important thing to accomplish in treating acute pancreatitis is to immediately remove the offending agent if possible, and to then provide the standard kinds of support: intravenous fluids, electrolyte replacement, and analgesia, for example. The vast majority of cases of acute pancreatitis are mild and will respond positively to treatment. Some of the dangerous complications of the condition, though, include pancreatic pseudocyst, fistula formation, hypocalcemia, renal failure, pleural effusion, and sepsis.

Chronic pancreatitis

Introduction and symptoms -- Chronic pancreatitis is irreversible parenchymal destruction that will eventually result in pancreatic dysfunction. This condition manifests as frequent episodes of severe pain. Individuals are more likely to suffer from chronic pancreatitis if they also have alcoholism, gallstones, hyperparathyroidism, or congenital malformation. An individual suffering from chronic pancreatitis is likely to report recurrent instances of epigastric pain, anorexia, nausea, constipation, flatulence, steatorrhea, and diabetes mellitus. A positive diagnosis of the condition can be made when laboratory tests indicate elevated or normal amylase and lipase, as well as glycosuria, pancreatic calcifications, and a mild ileus that is evident on a CT or abdominal X ray.

Diagnosis and treatment -- The treatment for chronic pancreatitis includes measures aimed at calming the symptoms as well as measures aimed at eliminating the cause of the disorder. A typical regimen includes analgesia, exogenous lipase or trypsin and a medium-chain fatty acid diet, a general avoidance of causative agents, celiac nerve block, and any surgery that is necessary for intractable pain or structural causes. Recovery from this condition is quite possible, although many individuals will continue to suffer from chronic pain, pancreatic exocrine, and endocrine dysfunction. Some of the more worrisome complications that can develop out of chronic pancreatitis are chronic pain, malnutrition and weight loss, and pancreatic cancer.

Pancreatic cancer

Introduction and symptoms -- The vast majority of instances of pancreatic cancer are pancreatic head adenocarcinomas. Individuals are much more likely to develop pancreatic cancer when they smoke, have chronic pancreatitis, have a relative with pancreatic cancer, or consume a high amount of fat in their diet. Demographically, pancreatic cancer is particularly common among men in their 60s. Patients with pancreatic cancer will typically present with abdominal pain that radiates towards the back; other common complaints include jaundice, a lack of appetite, nausea, vomiting, weight loss, fatigue, weakness, and indigestion. A thorough physical examination often will indicate that the patient has a palpable but non-tender gallbladder (this is known as Courvoisier's sign) or migratory thrombophlebitis (known as Trousseau's sign).

Diagnosis and treatment -- In order to diagnose pancreatic cancer, one should perform a CT scan in order to detect pancreatic masses, dilated pancreatic and bile ducts, metastases, and the extent of vascular involvement. In cases where a mass cannot be visualized, it may be necessary to perform an endoscopic ultrasound or endoscopic retrograde cholangiopancreatography. Some patients may even require fine-needle aspiration in order to get a full visualization. As for treatment, most patients will present with metastatic disease and so treatment will be palliative. Oftentimes, pancreatic head tumors will be found that display no evidence of metastization, and so it will be possible to resect using what is known as the Whipple procedure also known as pancreaticoduodenectomy.

Gynecological Disorders

Breast cancer

Introduction and etiology -- Breast cancer is the leading form of cancer in women, occurring in one out of nine, and the second highest cause of death from cancer, following lung cancer. Breast cancer can affect men as well. While breast cancer often happens in patients who have none of the known risk factors, there are several that can be outlined. Some risk factors are genetic, such as having a first-degree relative suffer from breast cancer, while others are due to lifestyle choices, such as smoking or having a low-fiber and high-fat diet. Increased estrogen is also a cause, as are age, BRCA1 and BRCA2 mutations, and having no children or children after 35. 45% of breast cancer occurs in the upper outer quadrant of the breast, 15% happens in the upper inner quadrant, 5% in the lower inner quadrant, 10% in the lower outer quadrant, and 25% in the subareolar area.

Symptoms -- Patients often feel a lump through self-examination, and it is recommended to women over 40 that they undergo mammograms for the purpose of revealing breast cancer. Early findings might be a single, painless, vague mass, and later findings could be breast enlargement, redness, pain, nipple or skin retraction, swollen axillary glands, or fixation of mass to the skin or chest wall. Late findings include edema of the arm, swollen lymph nodes, ulceration, metastases to the bone, lung, and liver. Once the breast cancer has reached the state of a metastatic disease, there can be bone pain, jaundice, weight loss, a firm axillary node larger than 1 cm, axillary nodes that are fixed to the skin, or ipsilateral supraclavicular or infraclavicular nodes. Breast cancer has four stages: stage I, with tumors smaller than 2 cm, stage II, with tumors between 2 and 5 cm, stage III, where the axillary nodes are involved, and stage IV, in which there are distant metastasis.

Diagnosis -- With a mammography, higher density with microcalcifications and irregular borders can be detected. An ultrasound can be used to identify a solid mass, as opposed to a benign cyst. Use tumor markers, in recurring cases, of CEA and CA 15-3 or CA 27-29. The receptor status of the tumor can be found by determining estrogen receptor, progesterone receptor, and HER2/neu position. For Stage IV, perform a bone scan and a CT of the chest, abdomen, pelvis, and brain to find any present metastases. A CXR will check for pulmonary metastases, and perform labs to look for higher EST, higher alkaline phosphatase, and increased levels of calcium.
In half of patients with stage IV breast cancer, there will be pleural effusion, which causes chest pain and painful breathing. Edema of the arm is also a typical complication.

Treatment -- For patients who are estrogen receptor negative, administer chemotherapy. Prescribe tamoxifen for all hormone receptor positive patients, and for HER2/neu-expressive cancers, trastuzumab is very effective. A partial mastectomy with partial axillary dissection, followed by chemotherapy, or a modified radical mastectomy are two surgical options. If there is the tumor is large, in a subareolar location, fixed to the chest wall, involves the nipple or overlying skin, or there are multifocal tumors, the breast must undergo a total mastectomy. In stage IV, begin treatment with radiotherapy and hormone therapy, with a mastectomy if necessary for removing the tumor(s). If the cancer is restricted to the breast, there is 75—90% cure rate. Once it spreads to the axilla, the rate drops to a five-year survival rate of 40—50%. If the patient is ER- or PR-positive, this is encouraging. However, aneuploidy, having one or a few chromosomes above or below the normal number, is an unfavorable factor.

Breast disease

Fibrocystic breast disease -- Caused by an exaggerated stromal tissue response to hormones and growth factors, this disease most often occurs in women between the ages of 30 and 50 and is connected to trauma and caffeine use. The patient may have painful, often multiple masses in both breasts, sometimes accompanied by nipple discharge. The size of the masses often fluctuates quickly, and pain and mass size increase while patient is premenstrual. To diagnose, perform a needle biopsy or excisional biopsy. The chance of breast cancer is raised if there is either ductal epithelial hyperplasia or cellular atypia. There is no real treatment.

Fibroadenoma -- Fibroadenoma is the primary breast lesion found in women younger than 30. It is a benign and slow-growing breast tumor and has epithelial and stromal factors. A large fibroadenoma is known as cystosarcoma phyllodes. It is a mass 1—5cm in diameter, and is round, fairly mobile, and not tender. Use a breast ultrasound, needle biopsy, or FNA to diagnose. The tumor can be removed, though they often reoccur.

Dysmenorrheal

1st degree dysmenorrheal -- Also known as menstrual cramps, is caused by contractions of the uterus during expulsion of unneeded contents and by the passage of clotted menstrual blood through the cervix. This usually occurs in the first or second day of the menstrual cycle. It will begin during the first year or two of menstruation, and the level of pain may increase with age. While there are no pathologic findings on a pelvic exam, the patient will present with cramping pain in the pelvic area, which often affects the back or inner thighs. A patient might also experience nausea, diarrhea, flushing, or headaches. Pain relievers and for some women, exercise, can be reduce the symptoms. Oral contraceptives can be prescribed and decrease the severity of menstrual pain through ovulation suppression.

2nd degree dysmenorrheal – Occurs when menstrual pain have an organic cause, such as PID or endometriosis.

Contraception

There are many forms of contraception, each with its own advantages and disadvantages. Some rely on behavior, such as the highly ineffective coitus interruptus, and the rhythm method, in which coitus is avoided during times of fertility that have been predicted through body temperature and vaginal discharge. Hormonal methods include Depo-Provera, which is a series of shots over the course of several months and Levonorgestrel, which is an implant. More hormonal methods are the prescription oral contraceptive pills, which are a combination of estrogen and progestin and must be taken every day, progestin-only pills, which are not as effective as oral contraceptives but can be used by lactating women, and the birth control patch, which is affixed to the skin. Emergency contraception, known as the morning-after pill, is a high-dose of OCP that can be taken up to 72 hours after unprotected sex and is not available OTC.

Barrier methods consist of condoms, diaphragms and cervical caps, which must be obtained through a physician, and IUDs, which must be inserted by a physician and can lead to uterine perforation, infection, ectopic pregnancy, and higher risk of PID. The only form of contraception that also provides protection against STDs is the condom. The two forms of permanent, surgical contraception are tubal ligation, in which the woman's fallopian tubes are severed and secured, and vasectomy, in which a man's Vas Deferens is cut. Some of the factors that prevent a woman from using oral contraceptives are pregnancy, breast cancer, history of thromboembolic disorders, stroke or CAD, tumor of the liver, estrogen-dependent cancer, and smoking cigarettes. Nor should a woman use an IUD if she is pregnant, has a history of PID, or is suffering from a gynecological infection or abnormal vaginal bleeding.

Amenorrhea

1st degree amenorrhea -- Girls usually start menstruating at puberty, and the failure for this to happen is called amenorrhea. If a girl has not menstruated by age 16 and has no sexual characteristics by age 14, it is 1st degree amenorrhea.

1st degree amenorrhea can be the result of Mullerian anomalies, vaginal agenesis, or an imperforate hymen, which all occur with normal levels of FSH. Other causes are high levels of LH, which result in testicular feminization, and high levels of FSH, causing ovarian failure or gonadal dysgenesis. It also happens because of steroidogenic enzyme defects or constitutional development delay, the result of low or even normal FSH levels. Low or normal FSH can also cause hypothalamic dysfunction, such as anorexia, weight loss, stress, tumor, or Kallmann's syndrome, and primary pituitary dysfunction. To treat hypothalamic amenorrhea, give the patient gonadotropins to induce ovulation. If caused by a tumor, it should be removed. For women with premature ovarian failure under 40, prescribe estrogen and progestin, or just progestin if the patient had a hysterectomy.

If a female stops menstruating for three consecutive months after having normal menses, it is 2nd degree amenorrhea. While the primary cause of 2nd degree amenorrhea is pregnancy, due to higher levels of beta-hCG, there are other causes as well. Those caused by lower or normal levels of FSH are hypothalamic dysfunction, caused by stress, anorexia, over-exercise, pituitary dysfunction, such as Sheehan's syndrome or panhypopituitarism, and hyperprolactinemia. High levels of FSH cause premature ovarian failure, 1st degree hypogonadism before 40, and menopause. Low or normal levels of FSH can lead to PCOS, and normal FSH can result in Asherman's syndrome (often caused by endometritis or postpartum scarring) and cervical stenosis.

Endometriosis

Endometriosis is a non-cancerous condition in which the body produces tissue that looks like endometrial tissue in abnormal places, particularly in the abdomen and dependent parts of the pelvis and ovaries. While a patient will often exhibit no symptoms, 2nd degree dysmenorrhea is one symptom of this condition. Women may also suffer from dyspareunia, which is painful intercourse, infertility, and rectal pain with bleeding. A laparoscopy should be performed to determine if a patient has endometriosis or PID. Classic lesions are blue-black or dark brown in appearance. An ultrasound can distinguish complex, fluid-filled masses from neoplasms and an MRI can be used to detect submucous myomas and adnexal masses. Prescribe GnRH analogs, danazol, or combination oral contraceptives to repress ovulation for 4 to 9 months, preventing cyclic stimulation of endometrial implants. For more severe cases, surgery is suggested.

Premenopausal uterine bleeding

In the case of abnormal uterine bleeding, in which blood loss is higher than the mean average 40mL in normal menses, compare the current menses cycle to that of the last menstrual period. In menorrhagia, which can cause anemia, blood loss will be more than 80mL in a cycle, and the flow will last more than 8 days. This can be a sign of another disease, such as uterine cancer or fibroids, or a hormonal disorder. If the length of time between cycles increases to between 35 and 90 days, this is oligomenorrhea—less bleeding than usual. Polymenorrhea is frequent menstruation on an under-21 day cycle and is anovular. Bleeding between periods is called metrorrhagia, and menometorrhagia is excessive and irregular bleeding. Both can cause anemia and may be signs of an underlying problem. While ovulation bleeding occurs in a typical menstrual cycle, anovulatory bleeding is dysfunctional uterine bleeding, caused by levels high levels of estrogen that are not counterbalanced by adequate levels of progesterone.

Postmenopausal uterine bleeding

If there is vaginal bleeding for six months or more after the menstrual function stops, it is considered to be cancer until another proven cause is found. Most women will have painless uterine bleeding, and vulvar or vaginal bleeding, ulcers, or neoplasms are possible. A PAP smear should be performed, as well as a transvaginal ultrasound. This is to measure the endometrial thickness, with more than 4 mm indicating the need for an endocervical curettage and endometrial aspiration to rule out cancer or hyperplasia. To treat simple or complex endometrial hyperplasia, which can be precancerous, the patient should undergo cycle progestin therapy and a repeat D&C or biopsy. If necessary, perform an aspiration curettage to remove the offending cells. If there is endometrial hyperplasia with atypical cells or carcinoma, a hysterectomy should be performed. Endometrial cancer may develop.

To diagnose this problem, perform labs for beta-hCG, CBC, and ESR. Always do a pregnancy test, since that is the highest cause of abnormal bleeding. If the patient has ovulatory bleeding, then check for cervical masses, perform a hysteroscopy and get a biopsy if needed.

For anovulatory bleeding, perform a PAP smear, order TFTs, perform an ultrasound to check for ectopic pregnancy or adexal masses, get an MRI to diagnose myomas and adenomyosis, and for women older than 35, get an endometrial biopsy. Progestins will stabilize endometrial growth, and combination OCPs will help active bleeding. If the bleeding is heavy, danazol, estrogen, GnRH agonists or OCPs should be prescribed. For menorrhagia, NSAIDs will bring down the blood loss.

Polycystic ovarian syndrome (PCOS)

Also known as Stein-Leventhal syndrome, this is a frequently occurring endocrine disorder in reproductive women. Symptoms include amenorrhea or irregular menstruation, hirsutism in 70% of cases, obesity in 40%, virilization in 20%, and often infertility. Women with this disorder do not ovulate every month and are at higher risk for high blood pressure, diabetes, heart disease, and endometrial cancer, though this can be combated through exercise and weight loss. HAIR-AN syndrome is a form of PCOS characterized by hyperandrogenism, insulin resistance, acanthosis nigricans. To diagnose, check for a high LH/FSH ratio, high testosterone (total +/-free), and perform an ultrasound to check ovaries for small cysts that are characteristic of this disorder. Different pharmaceuticals can induce menstruation, which may treat infertility and reduce the risk of cancer, and treat acne and hirsutism.

Hirsutism and virilization

Hirsutism is the presence of excessive facial and bodily hair. Virilization is defined as excessive androgenic influence. A patient can suffer from an overabundance of hair on the chin, upper lip, abdomen, and chest. It is also quite possible for a patient to have acne, a deep voice, be balding, have increased strength, clitoromegaly, and amenorrhea. Increased androgens, with testosterone higher than 2ng and DHEAS higher than 7 micrograms/mL, require an adrenal or ovarian tumor to be ruled out. If the patient has increased serum testosterone, an ovarian tumor is likely. Higher levels of DHEAS are probably the result of an adrenal problem, such as a tumor, Cushing's syndrome, or congenital adrenal hyperplasia. Once the cause of the hirsutism or virilization has been pinpointed, then treatment of that cause should decrease the original problem.

Infertility

Infertility is the inability to conceive despite repeated unprotected intercourse. Men and women can be infertile, but most often the male partner is the source. 40% of cases are abnormal spermatogenesis (low sperm count and motility), 30% are anovulation, 20% are female anatomic defects, and 10% are of unknown cause. The causes of male infertility can be testicular injury or infection, medications, and thyroid or liver disease. To diagnose, perform a semen analysis and check prolactin. To treat male infertility, intrauterine insemination, donor insemination, and IVF are all options. For women, infertility can be the result of old age, previous STDs, abortions, pregnancies, and abnormal menstrual cycles. The basal body temperature should be checked to evaluate ovulation, and perform labs to look for other causes. Clomiphene may help, as can tubal or uterine surgery, GnRH analogs, and IVF. Adoption is also a viable option for many couples looking to conceive.

Menopause

Most often occurring at age 51, menopause is the time when there has been no menstruation for 12 consecutive months due to the stopping of follicular development. There are many symptoms, some remembered through "menopause wreaks HAVOC: Hot flashes, Atrophy of the Vagina, Osteoporosis, Coronary heart disease," with others being insomnia, anxiety or irritability, vaginal bleeding, mood changes, loss of libido, dyspareunia, forgetfulness, and night sweats. High levels of FSH and LH can confirm this change, as can a DEXA scan for osteoporosis, a vaginal cytologic exam, and a lipid profile. Hormone replacement therapy can combat symptoms, though long-term use is dangerous and is not possible for some patients. To treat vaginal atrophy, vaginal cream can help, and if it is a long-term problem, prescribe an estradiol vaginal ring. Osteoporosis can be combated with calcium supplements and exercise.

Ectopic pregnancy

An ectopic pregnancy occurs when a fertilized egg settles outside of the uterus. 95% of cases are in the Fallopian tube, but they may also happen in the ovary, cervix, and abdominal cavity. Among the risk factors are a history of PID, prior ectopic pregnancy, IUD use, endometriosis, a history of repeated induced abortions, and tubal or pelvic surgery. The first symptom is usually pain, which might be pelvic, abdominal, or even felt in the shoulder or neck. If a pregnant woman in the first trimester exhibits amenorrhea with light vaginal bleeding and lower abdominal/pelvic pain, she likely has an ectopic pregnancy. 75% of patients will have abnormal uterine bleeding, 50% will have secondary amenorrhea, and 33% will have dizziness and light-headedness from internal bleeding. A ruptured Fallopian tube must usually be surgically removed, and patient may have sudden, sharp abdominal pain and tachycardia

A pelvic exam to test for pain, tenderness, and abdominal mass or labs testing for high beta-hcG can be used to diagnose. An ultrasound that reveals an empty uterus with a beta-hCG of 6500 mIU/mL is a high indication of an ectopic pregnancy. To treat an ectopic pregnancy, expectant management can be used for asymptomatic patients with low beta-hCG titers and a low risk of rupture. Methotrexate will work for less than 3-cm, unruptured ectopic pregnancies in asymptomatic women. Surgical options are salpingostomy, in which the tube is incised and only the fetus removed, salpingectomy, entire tube removal, and salpingo-oophorectomy, with both the tube and ovary removed. The fetus will always be lost in an ectopic pregnancy, and the mother may be as well. Other complications include hemorrhagic shock, infertility, future ectopic pregnancy, and Rh sensitization.

Cervicitis

Cervicitis is the inflammation of the uterine cervix (the canal that connects the uterus to the vagina). The causes, the most common of which are infectious, are *Chlamydia*, gonococcus,

Trichomonas, herpes simplex virus, and human papilloma virus, with the noninfectious causes being radiation exposure, trauma, and malignancy. A patient may present with a yellowish mucopurulent discharge, cervical motion tenderness, and no other signs of pelvic inflammatory disease. A positive diagnosis of cervicitic can be made after a biopsy confirms the presence of infectious cause. The usual treatment for cervicitis includes antibiotics and erythromycin.

Vaginitis

Vaginitis is a common gynecological condition, caused by the decrease of *lactobacillus*, which prevents the growth of harmful organisms in the vagina by causing slight acidity. Various causes are feminine hygiene products, medications, sexually transmitted diseases, intercourse, and stress, all of which can change the normal vaginal pH and lead to pathogens replacing *lactobacillus*. Women with diabetes develop vaginitis more often than women without diabetes. Patients will often present with itching, burning, pain and abnormal discharge. Check with patient about the last menstrual period, recent sexual activity, and use of oral contraceptives, tampons, or douches. To diagnose, check pH level of discharge, a urine sample to rule out a UTI, and treat with antifungal vaginal cream or oral medication.

Pelvic inflammatory disease

Introduction, symptoms and diagnosis -- In pelvic inflammatory disease, the upper genital tract will suffer a polymicrobial infection associated with *Neisseria gonorrhoeae* in one-third of cases, *Chlamydia trachomatis* in one-third of cases, and endogenous aerobes/anaerobes. Among the risk factors are non-Caucasian ethnicity, douching, smoking, prior pelvic inflammatory disease, and the use of intrauterine devices. A positive diagnosis of pelvic inflammatory disease can be made after laboratory tests indicate a white blood cell count above 10,000 and an elevated erythrocyte sedimentation rate. A saline microscopy may indicate cervical or vaginal discharge.

Treatment and complications -- Patients who are believed to have pelvic inflammatory disease should be given antibiotics even before the diagnosis is fully confirmed. The antibiotic regimens are cefotoxin with probenecid for one dose (regimen A); intramuscular ceftriaxone once and doxycycline for two weeks (regimen B); and ofloxacin for two weeks and metronidazole for two weeks (regimen C). Patients should be given intravenous antibiotics if they are suspected to have some other condition, like appendicitis, or if they are pregnant. If a patient is discovered to have a turbo-ovarian abscess, then it should be excised surgically. Some of the dangerous complications of pelvic inflammatory disease include recurrent infection, ectopic pregnancy, and infertility.

Endometrial cancer

Endometrial cancer, or cancer of the inner lining of the uterus, occurs most often in postmenopausal women. This is due to some connection between excess amounts of estrogen and the occurrence of endometrial cancer. Patients with endometrial cancer will present with vaginal bleeding. The positive diagnosis of endometrial cancer can be made after an endocervical biopsy; the Pap smear is not effective in diagnosing this kind of cancer. Treatment usually includes a total abdominal hysterectomy and bilateral salpingo-oophorectomy, along with dissection of the lymph nodes. This form of adenocarcinoma can usually be prevented by taking progesterone to counterbalance estrogen and maintaining a healthy weigh through a low-fat diet.

Toxic shock syndrome

Toxic shock syndrome is a life-threatening illness typically found in menstruating women who are suing tampons. The toxin contracted from prolonged use of a tampon can lead to bullous impetigo, scalded skin syndrome, and enterotoxin food poisoning. Individuals who are suffering from toxic shock syndrome will present with nausea, high fever, vomiting, and low blood pressure that can quickly lead to shock. Occasionally, a patient with toxic shock syndrome will present with a diffuse erythematous macular rash. The diagnosis of toxic shock must be based on clinical impression, as the blood culture will be negative. The source of the toxin should be immediately removed, and the patient should be given a massive infusion of fluids. Also, if the infection is found to be due to staphylococcus, the patient should be given nafcillin or oxacillin.

Vulvar cancer

Vulvar cancer typically occurs in postmenopausal women who have had a long period of vulvar irritation with pruritus and genital warts. Women are particularly at risk of developing vulvar cancer when they have the human papilloma virus. A physical examination may indicate a condition resembling chronic vulvar dermatitis, or a large ulcerated area in the vulva. Biopsy may be performed in order to obtain a positive diagnosis. If the cancer remains in situ (that is, if it has not spread to other parts of the body), then it should be surgically excised. If it has become an invasive cancer, then either a radical vulvectomy and regional lymphadenectomy or an excision of the tumor and a dissection of the inguinal lymph node should be performed.

Cervical cancer

Cervical cancer is especially common among women who began having sex before the age of 18 and have had many sexual partners. Typically, the women afflicted with cervical cancer are premenopausal. Though cervical cancer is often asymptomatic, it may present with bleeding after sex, metrorrhagia, and a bloody or purulent discharge. A thorough physical examination will reveal bladder and rectal dysfunction and cervical ulceration. A positive diagnosis is confirmed by a Pap smear. If the disease is caught early, the patient may be given radiotherapy, lymphadenectomy, and a radical hysterectomy. If the disease is more advanced, she may be given radiation or chemotherapy. Women are at greater risk of cervical cancer if the have the human papilloma virus.

Fibroids

Fibroids, otherwise known as uterine leiomyoma, are common benign tumors of the uterus. Often asymptomatic, these tumors can also lead to problems like heavy or extended menstrual bleeding, pelvic pain, and reproductive dysfunction. A positive diagnosis of fibroids can be made after a complete blood count indicates anemia, and an ultrasound indicates uterine myomas. The ultrasound may also be used to confirm that ovarian cancer is not present. The treatment for fibroids will include emergent surgery as it is required. Women who are still able to bear children should receive myomectomy, while postmenopausal patients may be better served by a total or subtotal abdominal/vaginal hysterectomy. As for medication, bleeding can be stemmed with danazol or medroxyprogesterone acetate.

Ovarian cancer

Ovarian cancer is a malignant tumor of the ovary, the egg sac of a female. This kind of cancer usually occurs in postmenopausal women above the age of fifty. Though ovarian cancer may not have any symptoms at all, it also may present with bloating, gastrointestinal disorders, and thrombophlebitis. A more thorough physical examination may reveal a palapable adrenal mass, pedal enema, and ascites. A positive diagnosis of ovarian cancer can be made after an ultrasound or abdominal CT scan indicates a mass. The normal treatment for ovarian cancer is a total abdominal hysterectomy in combination with bilateral salpingo-oophorectomy; chemotherapy may also be recommended in some cases. The use of oral contraceptives has been shown to decrease the instance of ovarian cancer.

Renal, Urinary, Male Reproductive Systems

Hypernatremia

Introduction and symptoms -- Hypernatremia is an elevated level of sodium in the blood, defined as more than 145 mEg/dL. This condition is typically the result of dehydration, although it can also be caused by certain medications. Patients with this problem will typically present with thirst, oliguria or polyuria. Some of the alterations in mental state that can occur as a result of hypernatremia are anxiety, confusion, and personality change. Patients may experience focal deficits or seizures in extreme cases. An examination of a patient suffering from hypernatremia will reveal doughy skin and some of the symptoms of depleted volume. The various causes of hypernatremia can be summarized as the 6 Ds: diuretics, dehydration, diabetes ensipidus, doctors (that is, from iatrogenic causes), diarrhea, and disease.

Diagnosis and treatment -- A positive diagnosis of hypernatremia is based on a clinical exam and an assessment of urine volume and osmolality. If the patient is suffering from hypernatremia as a result of pure water loss, then this is probably due to nephrogenic diabetes (that is, diabetes originating in the kidneys). Patients with this sort of hypernatremia will pass large amounts of extremely diluted urine. Patients who are suffering from hypernatremia because of hypertonic gains in sodium may be doing so because of elevated levels of aldosterone. Other patients are suffering from hypotonic fluid loss as a result of diminished fluid intake, renal disease, diuretics, or diarrhea. The treatment of hypernatremia should focus on the underlying causes; hypotonic saline, D5W, or water may be administered to restore proper volume. It is proper to slowly restore normal levels of hydration in order to avoid brain damage.

Enuresis

Enuresis, also known as urinary incontinence, can be caused by poor muscular tone, as well as by disorders of the kidneys, bladder, and ureter. Enuresis ranges from stress-induced, when certain position cause the involuntary passage of urine, to total, in which the patient is unable to contain any urine from exiting at any time. Urge incontinence is when the patient is overwhelmed by a sudden urge to urinate. Before enuresis is diagnosed, patients should receive a urinalysis and urine culture to exclude the possibility of urinary tract infection. The treatment for enuresis may include anticholinergic medications for urge incontinence; surgery for total incontinence; and corrective surgery for incontinence that is caused by stress.

Hyponatremia

Hyponatremia is a condition in which there is a significantly low level of sodium in the blood. Low sodium is defined as less than 136 mEq/L. This condition can be asymptomatic, or it can present as confusion, lethargy, nausea, and hyporeflexia. If left untreated, individuals with hyponatermia can fall into a coma and die. The degree of hyponatremia is classified by the osmolality of the urine. If the patient has high osmolality, then he or she will manifest hypertonic infusion and hyperglycemia; if the osmolality is normal, then the patient will demonstrate hypertriglyceridemia and paraproteinemia; if the osmolality is low, as in most cases, then the patient may be hypervolemic, euvolemic, or hypovolemic. The first two of these conditions are most commonly the result of renal failure, and can be treated by limiting the intake of water; hypovolemic individuals may be dehydrated and should be given saline infusions.

Hypokalemia

Hypokalemia is a significantly low level of potassium in the blood. This condition is often the result of excessive vomiting or the use of diuretics. A low level of potassium is defined as less than 3.6 mEq/L. Individuals suffering from hypokalemia will typically present with muscle weakness or cramps, or the obstruction of the intestines known as ileus. The ECG of an individual with hypokalemia will typically show a flattening of the T waves, and an extra wave after the T wave known as the U wave. There is usually an underlying case of hypokalemia that should be the focus of any treatment. Some patients may benefit from potassium supplements, while others may need magnesium in order to restore health.

Hyperkalemia

Hyperkalemia is an elevated amount of potassium in the blood. There are a few possible causes of this condition: overconsumption of potassium supplements, kidney failure, or certain medications. Significantly elevated potassium is defined as more than 5 mEq/L. This condition is often asymptomatic, though it may present with intestinal colic, paresthesias, weakness, and areflexia. The diagnosis of hyperkalemia is usually based on clinical impression, though it may be supported by repeat blood draws. It is typical for the electrocardiogram of an individual with hyperkalemia to display tall, jagged T waves. The treatment for hyperkalemia includes five major medications: insulin, calcium, bicarbonate, glucose, and kayexalate.

Hypocalcemia

Hypocalcemia is a significantly low level of calcium in the blood, clinically defined as less than 8.5 mg/dL. This condition can increase the sensitivity of the nervous system, resulting in tetany. Some of the etiologies of hypocalcemia are hypoparathyroidism, malnutrition, and acute pancreatitis. A patient with this condition will likely present with abdominal cramping, tetany, and perioral and acreal paresthesias. If an individual becomes chronically hypocalcemic, he or she will have soft bones and osteoporosis. In order to make a diagnosis of hypocalcemia, a doctor should have laboratory measures of calcium, magnesium, parathyroid hormone, albumin, and calcitonin. An electrocardiogram of an individual with hypocalcemia may indicate a prolonged QT interval. The treatment of this condition usually relies on the treatment of the underlying disorder, although some patients may benefit from oral or intravenous calcium.

Hypercalcemia

Hypercalcemia is a significantly elevated level of calcium in the blood. This is most often caused by hyperparathyroidism and cancerous malignancy. There are a number of nonspecific symptoms that may arise from hypercalcemia, including thirst, fatigue, nausea, and confusion. Individuals who have excessive levels of calcium can become weak and constipated, and may develop heart blocks. An elevated level of calcium is defined as more than 10.2 mg/dL. An electrocardiogram of a hypercalcemic individual may indicate a short QT interval. Hypercalcemia can be treated first with intravenous hydration, which makes the patient responsive to furosemide, a drug that increases the body's excretion of calcium. Patients should not be given thiazide diuretics, as these drugs tend to increase the body's intake of calcium.

Acute renal failure

Introduction and symptoms -- Acute renal failure is a sudden decline in the ability of the kidneys to perform their normal functions, resulting in excessive retention of blood urea nitrogen and creatinine. Oliguria, though commonly associated with renal failure, is not a necessary concomitant. There are three basic subtypes of renal failure. Intrinsic renal failure is caused by an injury within the kidney; prerenal failure is characterized by diminished renal perfusion; and postrenal failure is characterized by some obstruction to the outflow of urine, as for instance a kidney stone. Patients suffering from acute renal failure will present with uremic (excess urea in the blood) symptoms like malaise, confusion, and nausea. A closer physical examination will often indicate the presence of pericardial rub, asterixis, and hypertension.

Diagnosis and treatment -- A positive diagnosis of acute renal failure can be made after serum electrolytes and urine eosinophils have been measured. Prerenal failure is indicated by a fractional excretion of sodium less than 1%, a specific gravity greater than 1.02, or a blood urea nitrogen/creatinine ratio greater than 20. In order to treat acute renal failure, the patient should be given fluids or electrolytes as necessary, and may require dialysis. The indications that a patient is in need of immediate dialysis are organized in the mnemonic AEIOU: acidosis, electrolyte abnormalities, ingestions, overload, and uremic symptoms.

Hypomagnesemia

Hypomagnesemia is a significantly low level of magnesium in the blood, usually caused by either a low intake of the mineral or poor intestinal absorption of it. Low magnesium is defined as less than 1.5 mEq/L. It is very common for individuals suffering from hypomagnesemia to also be suffering from hypocalcemia and hypokalemia. Patients with this condition will present with anorexia, tetany (caused by the increases irritability of the nervous system), and muscle cramps and weakness. The diagnostic tests for hypomagnesemia are the same as those for hypocalcemia and hypoakalemia; an electrocardiogram will often show extended PR and QT segments. The treatment for hypomagnesemia may include oral/intravenous supplements of magnesium, although it should be noted that neither hypocalcemia nor hypokalemia can be resolved until magnesium deficiency is resolved.

Nephritic syndrome

Nephritic syndrome results from the inflammation of the glomerus, a minute round structure in the kidney made up of capillary blood vessels. Proteinuria often accompanies nephritic syndrome. The glomerus helps filter the blood during the production of urine, and so it is essential to the function of the kidneys. Patients suffering from nephritic syndrome, otherwise known as glomerulonephritis, will present with oliguria, brown-colored urine, and edema. A urinalysis will confirm the oliguria and possible proteinuria, and further laboratory tests should indicate diminished glomerular filtration rate along with increased amounts of blood urea nitrogen and creatinine. Patients with nephritic syndrome should be given corticosteroids to reduce the swelling of the glomerus; otherwise, the symptoms (uremia, hypertension, e.g.) should be the main focus of treatment.

Nephrolithiasis

Nephrolithiasis is the process through which a stone is formed in the kidney or lower down in the urinary tract. Besides stones made of calcium oxalate, patients may also develop stones made of uric acid, calcium phosphate, cystine, and struvite. The risk factors of nephrolithiasis include a family history of the disorder and low intake of fluids. Patients with this condition will present with a sudden attack of colicky flank pain; this pain may be severe enough to radiate to the genitalia. A urinalysis will indicate microscopic hematuria and a different urine pH. Patients who are suspected of having radiopaque stones should receive an abdominal X ray and/or renal ultrasound. Intravenous pyelography and noncontrast abdominal CT scans can also aid a diagnosis. The treatment for nephrolithiasis should include analgesia and hydration first, and then the doctor's attention needs to move to the passage of the stones. Stones that are less than 5 mm in diameter can probably pass through the urethra, while those less than 3 cm can be splintered by extracorporeal shock-wave lithotripsy.

Nephrotic syndrome

Nephrotic syndrome is a degenerative disease of the kidneys, in which the minute canals (tubules) that form the internal structure of the kidney are destroyed. Nephrotic syndrome manifests as proteinuria, generalized edema, hypoalbuminemia, and hyperlipidemia. Proteinuria is clinically defined as 3.5 or more grams per day. An individual suffering from proteinuria will typically present with generalized edema and foamy urine. A positive diagnosis of nephritic syndrome can be made after a urinalysis indicates lipiduria and proteinuria. Subsequent examinations of blood chemistry should indicate diminished levels of albumin and hyperlipidemia. In order to determine the underlying cause of the syndrome, a kidney biopsy should be performed. The treatment for nephritic syndrome combines salt and protein restriction with diuretic therapy and the diminution of angiotensin-converting enzyme inhibitors.

Polycystic kidney disease

Introduction and symptoms -- Polycystic kidney disease is when the kidneys become filled with scores of fluid-filled cysts. These growths diminish the effectiveness of the kidneys until the individual undergoes kidney failure. There are two types of this inherited disorder: autosomal dominant, which remains asymptomatic for a long period but becomes severe enough to require dialysis by age 60; and autosomal recessive, which is less common and results in almost immediate renal failure in children. Polycystic kidney disease will present as pain and hematuria, especially after the rupture of a cyst. Closer physical examination will often reveal hepatic cysts, hypertension, cerebral aneurysms, and mitral valve prolapse.

Diagnosis and treatment -- The diagnosis of polycystic kidney disease usually depends by means of an ultrasound, MRI, or CT scan that indicates numerous bilateral cysts located throughout the renal parenchyma, and it should be possible to note enlargement of the kidneys as well. The treatment of polycystic kidney disease is largely concerned with avoiding complications and avoiding the possibility of full-scale kidney failure. Renal cyst infections can be avoided in many cases by early detection and treatment of infections to the urinary tract. Patients who enter into end-stage renal dysfunction need to be given dialysis and, if possible, kidney transplantation. In dialysis, the body's blood is cleansed by a machine, bypassing the dysfunctional kidneys.

Ureteral reflux

Ureteral reflux occurs when urine moves backward from the bladder through the ureters to the kidneys. This condition is typically caused by the ureters not being properly attached to the submucosal bladder tissue, which makes the ureter incapable of impeding backwards urine flow during the contractions of the bladder. Ureteral reflux is suggested by a patient who presents with persistent urinary tract infections. In order to attain a positive diagnosis of the condition, a doctor should perform a voiding cystourethrogram. Infections of this kind need to be treated immediately; a mild reflux will resolve on its own with a minimum of antibiotic assistance. Very severe cases may require surgical ureteral implantation.

Renal tubular acidosis

The tubules are the tiny structures in the kidneys that filter the blood and help to produce urine. Renal tubular acidosis, then, is a net decrease in the secretion of H+ by the tubules or HCO-3 reabsorption, resulting in non-anion gap metabolic acidosis. The most prevalent form for renal tubular acidosis is Type IV, or distal renal tubular acidosis. In this type, the patient is suffering from a deficiency of aldosterone and therefore suffers an inability to reabsorb sodium, potassium, and hydrogen. The patient's urine pH in Type IV acidosis will be less than 5.3. This form of the disorder is most often caused by chronic kidney disease caused by diabetes, hypertension, or HIV. Patients should be given furosemide, fludrocortisone, and a diet that is low in potassium.

Diabetes insipidus

Introduction and symptoms -- Diabetes insipidus is a metabolic disorder in which the pituitary gland malfunctions, resulting in an increased output of urine and increased thirst. Diabetes insipidus can be either central or nephrogenic. In central diabetes insipidus, the posterior pituitary gland does not secrete the proper amount of the antidiuretic hormone, as a result of a tumor or a traumatic brain injury. In nephrogenic diabetes insipidus, the kidneys do not respond properly to the antidiuretic hormone. This form of diabetes insipidus is typically caused by renal disease and lithium medication. Patients with diabetes insipidus will present with hyper-urination, as well as a constant feeling of thirst. It is possible that individuals with this condition will be hypernatremic and dehydrated.

Diagnosis and treatment -- One common means of diagnosing diabetes insipidus is to deprive the patient of water and note the patient's excretion. This, of course, should not be done with patients who show signs of being dehydrated. Another way of diagnosing diabetes inspidus is to perform a desmopressin acetate challenge, in which patients are administered a close substitute for the antidiuretic hormone. Patients with diabetes mellitus will react with diminished urine output and increase urine osmolality, while patients with nephrogenic will not react in any significant way. The main goal of diabetes insipidus treatment is to remedy the underlying etiology; patients may also be given DDAVP through the nose if they have central DI, and placed on a low-salt, high-fluid program if they have neprogenic DI.

Benign prostatic hyperplasia

Introduction and symptoms -- Benign prostatic hyperplasia is a noncancerous condition in which the normal constituents of the prostate glans increase in size and number. This increase in prostatic mass can compress the urethra, making it difficult to urinate. By the age of 80, most men will suffer from benign prostate hyperplasia. If the enlarged prostate is obstructive, then the patient will complain of a constant feeling of bladder fullness without the ability to urinate satisfactorily. If the prostate is merely irritative, then the patient will complain of nocturia, daytime frequency, and opening hematuria. A digital rectal examination typically confirms the enlargement of the prostate; if the prostate is firm to the touch, the patient should be suspected of having prostate cancer.

Treatment -- Though most men over the age of 50 will develop benign prostatic hyperplasia, only a small percentage of these will need medical or surgical intervention. A positive diagnosis of the condition can be made after a digital rectal examination confirms the enlarged prostate and excludes the possibility of cancer. Infection and hematuria can be exluded after the performance of urinalysis and urine culture. Obstructive uropathy and renal insufficiency can be excluded by examination of the patient's creatinine levels. Most patients simply need to be monitored; more severe cases may benefit from the administration of alpha-blockers like terazosin, as well as 5alpha-reductase inhibitors like finasteride. Very serious cases may require surgical resection or open prostatectomy.

Inappropriate ADH secretion

Patients with inappropriate secretion of the antidiuretic hormone, also known as SIADH, may develop euvolemic hyponatremia because their release of the hormone is not osmotically stimulated. This condition is often associated with disorders of the central nervous system, like Hodgkin's disease, as well as with pulmonary disease and the antidepressant and antipsychotic medications. The positive diagnosis of inappropriate ADH secretion can be made after the patient's urine osmolality is found to be greater than 50-100 mOsm/kg at the same time that serum hyposmolarity exists. A subsequent test of the patient's urinary sodium levels confirms the diagnosis if it is greater than or equal to 20 mEq/L. The patient's fluid intake should be restricted and demeclocycline can be administered in order to manage the level of serum sodium.

Prostate cancer

Introduction and symptoms -- Prostate cancer is a major cause of death among men. Individuals are more at risk of prostate cancer as they advance in years and if they have a family member who has suffered from prostate cancer. All men over the age of 50 should receive an annual digital rectal exam to screen for prostate cancer. Prostate cancer usually begins asymptomatically, though patients may complain of some obstruction in their urination or of back pain caused by bone metastases. A digital rectal exam will discover a prostate that is enlarged and firm to the touch. It may even be possible to feel a hard nodule on the patient's prostate. If the patient's prostate is sensitive to the touch, it is likely that he or she has prostatitis.

Diagnosis and treatment -- The diagnosis of prostate cancer can be made after cancer cells are identified in a biopsy of the prostate. Cancer is also suggested when the patient has abnormally high levels of the prostate-specific antigen. Prostate tumors are scored on what is known as the Gleason histologic system; the two most abnormal samples are given a score from one to five, and these are combined to indicate the patient's overall level of cancer. The treatment for prostate cancer is more passive than for other forms of the disease, as prostate cancer often takes a very long time to develop. Very old patients may elect to have nothing done at all. Younger patients may opt for a radical prostatectomy or radiation therapy. If the growth appears to be metastasizing, then the patient can be given androgen ablation and chemotherapy.

Bladder cancer

Introduction and symptoms -- Bladder cancer is the most frequent malignant tumor that is found in the urinary tract. It is most common in men that have reached their 60s or 70s, and is usually a transitional cell carcinoma. Individuals are considerably more likely to develop bladder cancer when they have a diet rich in fat and meat, a schistosomiasis, are a smoker, or have been exposed to amiline dye. Patients with bladder cancer typically present with gross hematuria; unfortunately, though, bladder cancer is often asymptomatic until it is well advanced. The differential diagnosis for hematuria includes strictures, stones, infarction, inflammation, infection, tumor, tuberculosis, and trauma.

Diagnosis and treatment -- The positive diagnosis of bladder cancer depends primarily on cystoscopy performed on the growths taken during a bladder biopsy. A urinalysis performed on the patient will often indicate hematuria, while dysplastic cells may appear on cytology. An intravenous pyelography study is useful in examining the upper urinary tract. If the cancer remains in the bladder, then the patient can be treated with intravesicular chemotherapy. If the patient has an invasive form of bladder cancer that has yet to metastasize, then the patient should be given a radical cystectomy. If the patient has a superficial cancer, then he or she should be given a complete transurethral resection or intravesicular chemotherapy in combination with mitomycin-C. Large recurrent lesions require intravesicular chemotherapy.

Renal cell carcinoma

Renal cell carcinoma is an adenocarcinoma that originates in the tubules, the tiny passages that make up the bulk of the kidneys. The tubules help to remove toxins from the body. Renal cell carcinoma that occurs in children usually appears as Wilms' tumor. Individuals are at a greater risk of renal cell carcinoma if they smoke, are obese, or have acquired cystic kidney disease in end-stage renal disease. Patients suffering from renal cell carcinoma will typically present with hematuria (blood in the urine), palpable flank mass, and flank pain. Fever, anemia, and polycthemia are also potential symptoms. Renal cell carcinoma is diagnosed via ultrasound and/or CT scan, and is typically treated with surgical resection.

Cryptorchidism

Cryptorchidism is a disease in which one of the testicles fails to descend from the abdomen into the scrotum. If an individual does not have this condition corrected early in life, then he or she is at a greater risk of developing testicular cancer. Individuals who were born prematurely are at especial risk of cryptorchidism. A physical examination of a patient with this condition will find that the testicles cannot be digitally manipulated into position, though they can be palpated along the inguinal canal. The typical treatment for cryptorchidism is an orchiopexy, in which the testicle is brought down surgically. This procedure must be performed before the age of five in order to maintain the patient's fertility. Older patients may be treated with orthiectomy.

Testicular cancer

Testicular cancer is one of the most common cancers found in young men; they are typically discovered by the patient, and are especially common in those males with undescended testicles. Almost all forms of testicular cancer are malignant and derive from germ cells. Patients will typically present with nontender enlargement of the testes. A diagnosis of testicular cancer can be made after a testicular ultrasound confirms the presence of a mass. Doctors often use so-called tumor markers to monitor the progress of testicular cancer. Patients with this condition will typically have elevated levels of beta-human chorionic gonadotropin, and will often have elevated levels of alpha-fetoprotein. The treatment for testicular cancer may include the following: radical orchiectomy and radiotherapy/chemotherapy (especially for seminomas).

Erectile dysfunction

Erectile dysfunction is defined as the persistent inability to maintain the erection required for sexual intercourse. Erectile dysfunction is distinct from impotence caused by disease, injury, or drug use. One of the main obstacles to the treatment of erectile dysfunction is that patients will rarely seek treatment on their own. Erectile dysfunction may be either psychological or physiological; a complete patient interview and history must be obtained in order to determine the etiology of the disorder. If the patient is discovered to be having nocturnal erections, then psychological ED is implied. A diagnosis of physiological ED can be made when the patient's levels of testosterone and gonadotropin are found to be abnormal; in many cases, too, an elevated level of the hormone prolactin can diminish erectile function. Psychological impotence can be treated with psychotherapy; physiological ED can be treated with sildenafil or vardenafil, commercially known as Viagra and Levitra.

Pregnancy, Childbirth, Puerperium Disorders

Changes during pregnancy

Cervix, uterus, and vagina -- Both in response to the growing fetus and in order to prepare for the coming birth, the reproductive organs undergo a series of changes during pregnancy. The cervix undergoes softening and cyanosis approximately four weeks into a pregnancy. During or close to labor, there is a thick mucus clot in the cervical os that is expelled from the body. This is referred to as the "bloody show". The mucus is affected by progesterone, and when viewed microscopically, it will appear granular. At twelve weeks, the uterus palpates above the pubic symphysis. The vagina will emit violet-colored, thick acidic secretions. This is known as Chadwick's sign, and results from the increased blood flow to the vagina during pregnancy.

Endocrine system -- Pregnant women experience dramatic shifts in hormone production. The thyroid hormone experiences a higher thyroid-binding globulin, the result of increased estrogen levels. The active unbound hormone is not affected by the pregnancy, but the total and bound T3/T4 will go up. In order to maintain fetal glucose levels, human placental lactogen (HPL) will work as an insulin antagonist. This leads to postprandial hyperglycemia, fasting hyperinsulinemia/hypertriglyceridemia, and exaggerated starvation ketosis response. HPL can cause or worsen gestational diabetes. Total and free cortisol, which are produced by the fetal adrenal gland and the placenta, will both increase.

Cardiovascular -- In order to meet the expanded needs of a pregnant woman, the cardiovascular system makes some adjustments. The cardiac output is increased by 30—50% during pregnancy, while the heart rate goes up by 10—15 bpm, and stroke volume experiences a higher rate as well. The systemic vascular resistance (progesterone which contributes to smooth muscle relaxation) will be decreased. In the first trimester, blood pressure will go down. It will then achieve a nadir at 24 weeks and by the 40th week, should return to normal levels. Systolic murmur and audible S3 are normal during pregnancy, but a new diastolic murmur is abnormal. While pregnant, a patient's heart is displaced by the uterus upward and to the left, as is evident by a cardiomegaly on CXR.

Hematologic -- In order to sufficiently support the growing needs of the fetus, a pregnant woman's white blood count will increase all through a pregnancy to a mean of 10.5 million/mL, and can also increase during labor to more than 20 million/mL. The physiologic anemia is a result of unequal increase in plasma volume (50%) and red blood cell mass (30%), which leads to decreased hemoglobin and hematocrit. While the hemoglobin levels will go down, a hemoglobin of less than 11.0 mg/dL is never normal, and is probably caused by iron deficiency. Risk of deep venous thrombosis is at its highest in the puerperium, in hypercoagulable state. The primary nonobstetric cause of postpartum death is thromboembolic disease, also known as a pulmonary embolism.

Gastro-intestinal system and musculoskeletal -- Some of the more uncomfortable aspects of pregnancy are experienced in the gastro-intestinal system. Up to 70% of all pregnant women will experience nausea and vomiting. However, this is resolved between the 14th and 16th weeks as a result of the hCG rise leveling off. The decrease in gastroesophageal junction sphincter tone leads to an increase in acid reflux. As the large bowel motility decreases and the water resorption increases, the patient may experience constipation. There is a predisposition to gallstone formation from the increased biliary cholesterol saturation. As for the musculoskeletal system, a pregnant woman is likely to experience increased motility of the sacroiliac, sacrococcygeal, and pubic joints.

Renal and skin -- During pregnancy, the kidneys will dilate. This dilation of the collecting system might be mistaken for hydronephrosis, but is normal. The glomerular filtration rate will go up by 50%, and renal plasma flow will increase by 30%. The rennin-angiotensin system will be stimulated by the higher levels of estrogen and progesterone caused by pregnancy, while water retention and increased plasma volume are brought on by an increase of aldosterone. The epidermis will be affected by higher levels of estrogen, which may cause changes that resemble cirrhotic disease. Among these changes are palmar erythema, spider angiomas, and striae, which will appear on the breast, abdomen, and thighs. An increase in alpha-melanocyte-stimulating hormone and steroids will result in hyperpigmentation over the face (chloasma), midline (linea nigra), and perineum. There is also the possibility of diastasis recti, in which rectus muscles may separate in the midline. This will mean that some of the anterior uterus is covered only by skin, fascia, and peritoneum.

Pulmonary -- In the pulmonary system, a pregnant woman will experience an increase in tidal volume (V sub T) of 40%. There will also be a decrease in total lung capacity, residual volume, and expiratory reserve volume. The respiratory rate (RR) will be unaffected by the pregnancy and remain normal. There will be an increased minute ventilation (V sub T x RR), which will result in increased alveolar and arterial partial pressure of oxygen and decreased alveolar and arterial partial pressure of carbon dioxide. It is common for a pregnant woman to experience "dyspnea of pregnancy," which is probably the result of increased V sub T and decreased partial pressure of carbon dioxide.

Stages of labor

There are three basic stages of labor. In the latent part of the first stage, which begins with the onset of labor and ends at 4 cm dilation, the mother will begin to experience hypertonic uterine contractions. In the active part of the first stage, the mother will begin to experience prolongation along with cephalopelvic disproportion. This phase of labor lasts until dilation has become complete at about 10 cm. In the second stage of labor, the fetus will go through the cardinal movements; this stage lasts from the complete dilation of the cervix to the full delivery of the infant. In the third and last stage of labor, the placenta will separate and the uterus will contract, establishing homeostasis. This stage of labor ends with the delivery of the placenta.

Standard prenatal care

Every woman should gain weight during a pregnancy. For an average woman, the recommended weight gain is between 25 and 35 pounds. It shifts to 15 to 25 pounds for obese women, and then more for thin women. In addition to the weight gain, an extra 300 kcal/day is needed, and if a woman is breastfeeding, that should increase to 500 kcal/day for the duration of her lactation. As for nutrition, a pregnant woman should meet certain vitamin and mineral needs for the health of the fetus. It is important for a woman to have had 1 mg of folate daily for three months prior to conception and throughout the pregnancy. This is required to decrease the likelihood of neural tube defects. The need for iron is increased by both the needs of the fetus and by the expanding maternal blood supply. It is advised to add a supplement with 30—60 mg of elemental iron daily in the last half of the pregnancy. As a measure of precaution, prenatal vitamins are recommended throughout a pregnancy, although most needs can be achieved through diet.

Pregestational diabetes mellitus

There are both maternal and fetal complications of pregestational diabetes mellitus, which is caused by abnormally high levels of sugar in the blood and is diagnosed through blood sugar testing. Regular ultrasounds and a triple screen are necessary to check infant's GA and for abnormalities. Labor may need to be induced for the safety of mother and infant. The maternal complications are diabetic ketoacidosis, type 1 or hyperosmolar hyperglycemic nonketotic coma, type 2, preeclampsia or eclampsia, polyhydramnios, preterm labor, infection, cephalopelvic disproportion and need for C-section, postpartum hemorrhage, and maternal mortality. The fetal complications are macrosomia, cardiac and renal defects, hypocalcemia, polycythemia, neural tube defects, hyperbilirubinemia, intrauterine growth restriction, respiratory distress syndrome, hypoglycemia from hyperinsulinemia, birth injury, and perinatal mortality.

Gestational diabetes mellitus

Gestational diabetes mellitus occurs in almost five percent of all pregnancies, and is most likely to occur late in the term. This condition typically disappears after delivery. One of the dangerous complications of gestational diabetes is macrosomia, in which the baby grows abnormally large. This condition is usually asymptomatic, although an ultrasound may indicate that the fetus is larger than normal. The diagnosis can be confirmed if the patient has a fasting serum glucose level that is greater than 126 mg/dL. The best treatment for this condition is a strict monitoring of diet by the mother, and insulin injections if necessary. An occasional ultrasound may be useful in assessing the condition of the fetus.

Preeclampsia and eclampsia

During the third trimester, a patient might develop preeclampsia, which is a significant increase in blood pressure. Eclampsia is preeclampsia along with seizures. HELPP syndrome (Hemolysis, Elevated LFTs, Low Platelets) occurs in 25% of women with preeclampsia and eclampsia. Typical symptoms are malaise, nausea and/or vomiting, and pain in the upper abdomen. Some risk factors are black ethnicity, being younger than 20 or older than 35, nulliparity, multiple gestation, molar pregnancy, a family history of preeclampsia, renal disease, and chronic hypertension (also a risk factor in preeclampsia). This is diagnosed by urine analysis, protein discovered in the urine, CBC, electrolytes, amniocentesis (used to determine fetal lung maturity, which can allow for early delivery), uric acid, BUN/creatinine, LFTs, PT/PTT, fibrinogen and fibrin split products, ultrasound, and NST/CST/BPP. The only way to cure preeclampsia or eclampsia is to delivery the fetus, which should be done if this develops after 34 weeks or the mother is in danger.

Gestational and chronic hypertension

Gestational hypertension, once known as pregnancy-induced hypertension, is defined as the idiopathic hypertension without significant proteinuria, which is less than 300 mg/L. It begins in the second half of pregnancy, during labor, or within 48 hours postpartum. It is possible for a patient to later develop preeclampsia. Chronic hypertension occurs before conception and at less than 20 weeks' gestation. It may last for more than 12 weeks after delivery. It is treated by monitoring blood pressure and administering antihypertensives. Although they are used to treat other types of high blood pressure, it is important not to give ACEIs or diuretics because they can cause uterine ischemia, which causes complications that are like those caused by preeclampsia.

Teratogen drugs

There are several teratogen drugs, all of which will likely have an affect on the fetus, which is most susceptible in the organogenesis weeks (3—8). Alcohol can cause fetal alcohol syndrome, which always has microcephaly, midfacial hypoplasia, mental retardation, intrauterine growth retardation, and cardiac defects, and often causes hearing loss and frequent ear infections. Alcohol, when it doesn't cause FAS, can lead to alcohol-related neurodevelopmental disabilities. Cocaine use can lead to bowel atresias, intrauterine growth retardation, and microcephaly. Streptomycin can lead to cranial nerve VIII damage and ototoxicity. Tetracycline can result in small limbs, syndactyly, discolored teeth, and inhibited bone growth. Sulfonomides cause kerniceterus. Quinolines result in cartilage damage. Isotretinoin leads to heart and great vessel defects, deafness, and craniofacial dysmorphism. Iodide causes congenital goiter, mental retardation, and hypothyroidism.

Methotrexate use results in central nervous system malformations, intrauterine growth retardation, and craniofacial dysmorphism. Diethylsilbestrol use can cause clear cell adenocarcinoma of the vagina and cervix, genital tract abnormalities, and cervical incompetence. Thalidomide leads to limb reduction, cardiac and lung defects, pyloric or duodenal stenosis, ear and nasal anomalies, and gastrointestinal atresia. Coumadin results in stippling of bone epiphyses, intrauterine growth and mental retardation, and nasal hypoplasia. Lithium use leads to cardiac diseases, including Ebstein's anomaly. ACEIs can create fetal renal damage and oligohydramnios. Phenytoin can lead to nail hypoplasia, intrauterine growth and mental retardation, and neural tube defects. Carbamazepine creates fingernail hypoplasia, intrauterine growth and retardation, microcephaly, and neural tube defects. Valproic acid can cause neural tube defects as well as craniofacial and skeletal defects.

Oligohydramnios

When there is extremely low amniotic fluid (an amniotic fluid index of less than 5), that is known as oligohydramnios. If a rupture of membranes does not occur, oligohydramnios is 40 times more likely to result in perinatal mortality. It should be noted that if this is discovered, the overall well-being of the fetus should be checked. Among the causes are fetal urinary tract abnormalities, rupture of membranes, or chronic uteroplacental insufficiency. This is often asymptomatic or can be indicated by above average fundal height. To diagnose, test glucose for DM, perform a Rh screen, and use an ultrasound to check for fetal anomalies. Complications include preterm labor, fetal malpresentation, and cord prolapse.

Intrauterine growth retardation

Intrauterine growth retardation is characterized by extremely low fetal weight (below the 10th percentile) for the gestational age. If there is a discrepancy of more than 4 between fundal height (cm) and GA on exam, intrauterine growth retardation should be taken into consideration. This happens in between 3 and 7 percent of pregnancies. The two types of intrauterine growth retardation are symmetric (20%), occurring early in pregnancy and asymmetric (80%), happening late in a pregnancy. Assymetric may be caused by fetal problems, while symmetric is the result of maternal issues. Symmetric consists of low biparietal diameter, head and abdominal circumference, and femur length. The asymmetric cases only suffer from low abdominal circumference. It should be treated with steroids to aid in the lung development and possibly by an early delivery.

Rhesus Isoimmunization

Rhesus isoimmunization is caused by Rh-positive red blood cells entering the maternal bloodstream from the fetus through the placenta, inciting anti-RH IgC antibodies to form. When these antibodies then enter the placenta, it can result in hemolysis. Rhesus isoimmunization is usually the case in a second pregnancy, after the mother has already carried a Rh positive fetus and developed the antibodies, and thus quickly produces them again in memory plasma cells. Abortion and prior delivery of an Rh-positive infant are main causes of rhesus isoimmunization. On the initial visit, the mother should be tested for ABO and Rh blood groups and submitted to antibody screening. If negative, repeat screening at 26—28 weeks; if positive, check serially for high maternal anti-Rh IgC. In the fetus, it is found through amniocentesis or umbilical blood sampling, Coombs' titer, bilirubin levels, hematocrit, and reticulocytes.

To prevent fetal hemolysis, give Rh immune globulin if the mother is Rh-negative at 28 weeks and either the father is Rh-positive, his status is unknown, or paternity is unknown. If indeed the baby is Rh-positive, Rh immune globulin must also be given after the delivery. If the case is severe, delivery should be induced once fetal lungs have matured. Before delivering, intrauterine blood transfusions can correct a low fetal hematocrit. There are serious complications associated with this issue, such as fetal hypoxia and acidosis, kernicterus, prematurity, and death. It is also possible for hydrops fetalis to happen when hemoglobin drops to less than 7 g/dL, resulting in decreased protein and oncotic pressure, jaundice, high-output cardiac failure, and edema.

Polydramnios

A condition in which there is too much amniotic fluid, as defined by an amniotic fluid index of more than 20 via ultrasound. While this might happen in normal pregnancies, it is still quite possible for fetal chromosomal or developmental abnormalities to occur. Maternal diabetes mellitus, multiple gestation, isioimmunization, pulmonary abnormalities, fetal abnormalities such as anencephaly, and twin to twin transfusion syndrome are all causes of polydramnios. While there are often no symptoms, an exam might reveal greater than average fundal height. Use an ultrasound for fetal anomalies, glucose testing for diabetes mellitus, and an Rh screen to diagnose. The complications that can arise from this condition are cord prolapse, preterm labor, and fetal malpresentation.

Gestational trophoblastic disease

This disease is specific to women, and consists of one of two types of tumors: hydatidiform mole (benign) or choriocarcinoma (malignant). These tumors begin in the uterus after cancer cells grow in the tissues formed post-conception. Among the risk factors are being younger than 20 or older than 40, not having enough folate or beta-carotene in one's diet, and blood group (both of the woman and man). While 80% of GTD cases are hydatidiform mole (also referred to as a molar pregnancy), there is also the chance of an invasive mole at 10—15% and choriocarcinoma at 2—5%. Complete moles, paternally derived, are often caused by sperm fertilization of an empty ovum and have a chromosomal pattern of 46, XX. Incomplete moles happen when a normal ovum is fertilized by two sperm, often have a chromosomal pattern of 69, XXY and may contain fetal tissue.

The most common trait is first-trimester uterine bleeding, followed by hyperemedis gravidarum, preeclampsia or eclampsia, a uterine size greater than dates, and hyperthyroidism. There will not be a fetal heartbeat. A pelvic exam might show enlarged ovaries with bilateral theca-lutein cysts and/or expulsion of grapelike molar clusters into the vagina or blood in the cervical os. After treatment, cysts will be resolved. A significant increase in beta-hCG and a "snowstorm" appearance on a pelvic ultrasound indicate GTD. It is critical to identify the type of tumor, follow the beta-hCG, and prevent pregnancy for one year. Chemotherapy is required for a malignant tumor, and residual uterine disease should be treated with a hysterectomy. Complications consist of malignant GTD, pulmonary or central nervous system metastases, trophoblastic pulmonary emboli, and acute respiratory insufficiency.

Third-trimester bleeding

Third-trimester bleeding is defined as any bleeding after 20 weeks of gestation, and it complicates between 3 and 5% of pregnancies. It is generally caused by placental abruption and placenta previa. Among the other causes are bloody show, early labor, ruptured uterus, genital tract lesions and trauma. Placental abruption is the premature separation of an otherwise normal placenta and can be indicated by painful, dark vaginal bleeding, abdominal pain, and fetal distress. To diagnose, watch for retroplacental clot. The patient should be hospitalized and the fetus monitored; if it is a moderate or severe abruption, the fetus must be delivered—vaginally if mother and fetus are stable, or by C-section if they are not. Complications include hemorrhagic shock, coagulopathy with disseminated intravascular coagulation in 10%, and fetal hypoxia.

Placenta previa, defined as abnormal placental implantation, has three categories. They are total, in which the placenta covers cervical os, marginal, when the placenta extends to margin of os, and low-lying, with the placenta in close proximity to os. While there is rarely fetal distress, there will be painless, bright red bleeding which usually stops in an hour or two, with or without uterine contractions. The bleeding will most likely begin between 29—30 weeks. To diagnose, check for an abnormally positioned placenta and watch for transabdominal/transvaginal ultrasound sensitivity higher than 95%. Do not perform a vaginal exam. The patient with a premature fetus should be stabilized, fetal lung maturity must be assessed, and then delivery by C-section if there is persistent labor, life-threatened bleeding, fetal distress, or the gestational age is 36 weeks. Complications are placenta accrete, vasa previa, preterm delivery, premature rupture of membranes, intrauterine growth rate, and congenital anomalies.

Failure to progress

During labor and delivery, there can be problems which halt the process. In the first stage, there is a latent and active portion. In the latent part, failure to have progressive cervical change is categorized as prima, happening at more than 20 hours, and multi, happening at more than 14. To treat this problem, use therapeutic rest via parenteral analgesia, oxytocin, amniotomy, or cervical ripening. Active failure is when there is no progressive cervical change once 3—4 cm dilation has occurred. This can also be treated with amniotomy or oxytocin. If the patient does not respond, proceed with a C-section. The second stage is the arrest of fetal descent, with prima happening at more than 3 hours, and multi occurring at more than 2. Decrease the epidural rate, continue oxytocin to treat prima, and either perform an assisted vaginal delivery or a C-section in response to multi.

Preterm Labor

If labor begins between 20 and 37 weeks of gestation, it is preterm and makes up for 10% of the pregnancies in the U.S. While there are risk factors such as PROM, previous preterm labor or delivery, and placental abruption, most patients will not exhibit any risk factors. It is possible for a patient to have experienced cramps, lower back pain, pressure on her pelvis, and new vaginal bleeding or discharge. If there are regular uterine contractions of 3 or more lasting 30 seconds each over 30 minutes and concurrent cervical change past 37 weeks' gestation, a patient is experiencing preterm labor. Assess for contraindications to tocolysis, discount PROM through a sterile speculum exam, and use an ultrasound to assess fetus and amniotic fluid volume. The patient should be well-hydrated and put on bed rest, as well as given tocolytic therapy and steroids to boost fetal lung maturation. Give penicillin for strep if preterm delivery is imminent. Complications include respiratory distress syndrome, intraventricular hemorrhage, respiratory distress syndrome, bronchopulmonary dysplasia, and death.

Premature rupture of membranes

Before labor begins, these are called spontaneous rupture of membrane. Preterm PROM happens at more than 37 weeks, and a rupture at more than 18 hours before delivery is considered prolonged ROM. A distinguishing factor is the "gush" of clear or bloody amniotic fluid that most patients report, with or without uterine contractions. Check for pooling of amniotic fluid, a positive Nitrazine paper test and a positive fern test of amniotic fluid. Since this happens most often to women of low socioeconomic status, young mothers, smokers, and those with STDs, check for infections without doing a digital vaginal exam if the gestational age is under 34 weeks. Delay delivery with tocolytics if there appears to be no infection. In order to avoid infection, prescribe prophylactic antibiotics. Promotion of fetal lung maturity can be aided with corticosteroids. Give the patient antibiotics and induce labor if there is infection or fetal distress.

Caesarean section

When a vaginal birth is not possible, a caesarean section may be performed by surgically removing the infant through a division in the walls of the mother's abdomen and uterus. A C-section is probably necessary if the mother had a previous C-section, or has active genital herpes infection, cervical carcinoma, trauma, or is dead. Cephalopelvic disproportion is the number one reason for the performance of a C-section. They are also necessitated by placenta previa or placental abruption, a failed vaginal delivery, or post-term pregnancy. Fetal malposition, fetal distress, cord compression, and erythroblastosis fetalis all may require a C-section as well. The risk of a patient developing an endometrial infection increases after undergoing a C-section.

Fetal malpresentation

If a fetus does not present in vertex, with the head closest to the vagina, chin to chest, and an occiput anterior, it is a fetal malpresentation. It can be caused by prematurity, a prior breech delivery, hydrocephalus, and other factors. The most common malpresentation is breech, in which the fetal lower extremities or buttocks are presented into the mother's pelvis. In the frank breech (50—75%), knees are extended with thighs flexed, in a footling breech (20%), one or both legs are straightened below the buttocks, and a complete breech (5—10%) has knees and thighs flexed. Diagnose with Leopold maneuvers. Treat by leaving alone, since the vast majority of breeches will change to vertex by week 38. If this does not happen, try to turn the infant to vertex by applying pressure on the mother's abdomen. This may result in an emergency C-section. If the delivery is not preventable, use trial of breech vaginal delivery—cord prolapse and/or head entrapment may occur. An elective C-section is also possible, although not necessary.

Postpartum infections

A postpartum infection can be diagnosed once a patient has had a genital tract infection accompanied by a fever of 38 degrees Celsius or higher for at least two of the first ten postpartum days, discounting the first 24 hours. The most common infection is endometrial, in the inner layer of the uterus, which is more likely after a C-section. The symptoms of postpartum infection are endomyometritis, pneumonia or atelectasis (failure of the lung to expand at birth or a postpartum lung collapse), a urinary tract infection, pulmonary embolism or deep vein thrombosis, an episiotomy, mastisis or an abscess of the breast, and drug fever. Treatment consists of broad-spectrum IV antibiotics until the patient has been afebrile for 48 hours. If a patient doesn't respond to treatment after 48 hours, the problem could be septic pelvic thrombophlebitis, inflammation of a vein from a blood clot, or a pelvic abcess.

Postpartum hemorrhage

If before, during, or after delivering the placenta, a patient loses more than 500 mL of blood from a vaginal delivery, or more than 1000 mL of blood from a C-section, she is suffering a postpartum hemorrhage. There is a life-threatening possibility of acute blood loss, or anemia resulting from chronic blood loss. Another complication is Sheehan's syndrome, which is postpartum pituitary necrosis. Failure to lactate is the primary syndrome, resulting from decreased prolactin levels. The primary cause of postpartum hemorrhage (90%) is uterine atony, followed by genital tract trauma and retained placental tissue. Uterine atony can often be treated by a uterine massage, otherwise use an oxytocin infusion, methergine, or prostin. For genital tract trauma, surgery is necessary, while manually removing the placenta is possible for the retained placental tissue.

Mastitis

Known as mastitis, the inflammation of one or more mammary glands in the breast (most often in a lactating woman), this condition can be caused by either a mammary infection or a blocked milk duct. The breathing of S. aureus from the infant onto a damaged nipple also leads to mastitis. The symptoms typically show up 2—4 weeks after birth, and consist of focal breast tenderness, erythema, edema, warmth, and sometimes purulent nipple drainage. Ensure that it is not just breast engorgement by checking for a fever and increased white blood count. To treat mastitis, the woman should rest, apply warm compresses to the affected area, continue to breastfeed, and possible take antibiotics. If there is an abscess, it should be punctured and drained. Recurrent mastitis throughout nursing requires the consultation of a lactation expert.

Lactation and breast-feeding

Before the breast milk comes in, there is colostrum, which is high in protein, fat, secretory IgA, and minerals. The protective antibodies give the infant's immune system increased protection. The lactation process is kick-stared by delivery of the placenta, which decreases the levels of estrogen and progesterone that had been raised by the pregnancy. It is then perpetuated by breast-feeding, which stimulates the release of more prolactin and oxytocin, causing myoepithelial cell contraction and then the release of milk. Mature breast milk, containing fat, lactose, water, and protein, comes in within a week of giving birth. There are significant benefits to breast-feeding, both for the mother and the infant. It decreases the child's changes of developing allergies, increases weight loss for the mother, and helps the formation of the mother-child bond, encouraging a strong and healthy relationship. However, if a mother is HIV positive, has active hepatitis, or is on certain medications, she should not breastfeed.

Spontaneous abortion

If a fetus is lost before the 20th week, it is considered to be a spontaneous abortion (SAB). The majority of cases happen before the 16th week, and the majority of those cases occur before week 8. Around 20% of clinically recognized pregnancies will end in spontaneous abortion. Increased risks of spontaneous abortion are a history of incompetent cervix, loop electrosurgical excision procedure, DES exposure, an anatomically abnormal or injured cervix, chromosomal abnormalities in the fetus (first trimester), and various maternal factors in the second trimester. There are eight types of spontaneous abortion, many with similar forms of treatment. To diagnose a spontaneous abortion, check for lower levels of hCG, perform an ultrasound, determine maternal Rh type and give RhoGAM if it is negative, and keep all recovered tissue for analysis.

A complete SAB expels all products of conception (POC), and while there may still be spotting, pain will stop. An incomplete SAB expels some POC and leaves visible tissue in the vagina, accompanied by mild cramps and bleeding. A threatened SAB does not expel any POC—the fetus may be saved with bed rest and abstinence. This is accompanied by bleeding and possible abdominal pain. An inevitable SAB comes with uterine bleeding, cramps, and no likelihood of saving the fetus. A missed SAB does not expel POC, and there is no uterine bleeding. The pregnancy does not continue to develop, and its symptoms disappear, resulting in brownish vaginal discharge. A septic SAB has a maternal mortality of 10—15%, since there is endometritis that results in septicemia. A recurrent SAB is labeled as two or more consecutive SABs or three altogether. In this case, the patient should be checked for uterine and chromosomal abnormalities. Intrauterine fetal demise is the lack of fetal cardiac activity, the result of a small uterus for the GA.

Congenital hip dysplasia

Introduction and symptoms -- Congenital hip dysplasia is one of the more common birth defects; it is when the ball at the top of the thighbone is not well-suited to its socket. It is also possible for individuals with this condition to have loose or hyper-flexible ligaments in the hip joint. This dislocation of the femur heads is caused variously be poor development of the acetabulum because of poor musculature, or because of excessive uterine packaging during a breech birth (in which the buttocks, rather than the head, emerges first). The nature of the dislocation can be determined by performing Barlow's or Ortolani's maneuver, and the patient is likely to present with Alli's sign, in which his or her knees are at unequal heights.

Diagnosis and treatment -- Congenital hip dysplasia needs to be diagnosed early so that the child can be given a chance to develop normally. It can be helpful to perform an ultrasound if the child is older than ten weeks. If the child's hip makes a clicking noise when his or her legs are moved apart, this is indicative of congenital hip dysplasia. Also, the folds on the child's buttocks may be asymmetrical, and if the child is old enough to walk, he or she may walk with a limp. A radiograph is not helpful when the child is less than four months old due to the radiolucency of the neonatal femoral head. The most common treatment for congenital hip dysplasia is the Pavlik harness, which keeps the hip flexed and abducted. When this is ineffective, the leg may be placed in the proper position under anesthesia, and maintained there in a body cast.

SCFE

Slipped capital femoral epiphysis (SCFE) is a condition in which the growth plate of the femur is pushed out of position. This problem can result in hip pain, a stiff walking style, and occasional knee pain. This can be caused by some imbalance between the sex hormones and growth hormones. Individuals are considered to be especially at risk when they are obese, are between the age of 10 and 14, male, and of African-American heritage. Severe cases of SCFE will present with an inability to place weight on the afflicted leg. If a radiograph is taken of both hips in the anteroposterior and frog-leg lateral positions, then it will indicate posterior and medial displacement of the femoral head. The treatment protocol for SCFE should begin at once, and includes physical therapy and exercise. Obese individuals may need to lose weight

Legg-Calve-Perthes disease

Legg-Calve-Perthes disease is a hip disorder that is found in children, in which the blood supply to the head of the femur is interrupted. There is no known etiology for this disease, though it sometimes will occur in several members of the same family. The symptoms of the condition usually last less than a year and a half. These symptoms include pain in the hip and thigh, a limp, and a diminution in the size of the thigh. The patient is also likely to have limited abduction and internal rotation. In the period before the blood supply is reestablished, the bone is soft and more likely to fracture. If the patient has a full range of motion or if only part of the femoral head is involved, then he or she only needs to be monitored. If the condition is more serious, then bracing, hip abduction in a cast, or osteotomy may be recommended.

Ventricular septal defect

Ventricular septal defect is a hole in the wall that separates the lower chambers of the heart. This is the most common birth defect affecting the heart. This condition tends to transfer blood from the left to the right ventricle, which may fail under the increased load. If the defect is small, then it may be asymptomatic at birth; more serious defects may present with chronic respiratory infection, congestive heart failure, and failure to thrive. A closer physical examination will indicate a pansystolic murmur in the lower left sternal border; there will also be a pulmonic S2. An ECG is the best way to diagnose ventricular septic defect. Minor VSDs will resolve themselves, and large VSDs will require immediate surgical repair.

Osteosarcoma

Osteosarcoma is a cancer of the bone that particularly affects adolescents and young adults. It usually appears in the metaphyseal areas of the distal femur, proximal tibia, and proximal humerus. A patient with osteosarcoma will present unstoppable pain that is worse at night, and maybe with fever, weight loss, and night sweats. A closer examination may reveal erythema or enlargement over the location of the tumor. A positive diagnosis of osteosarcoma can be made after a radiograph indicates Codman's triangle, new bone formation at the diaphyseal end of the lesion). The osteosarcoma may also display a characteristic "sunburst pattern." The treatment for osteosarcoma includes chemotherapy and surgical procedures, all of which are aimed at preventing the necessity of amputation.

Atrial septal defect

Introduction and symptoms -- An atrial septal defect is a hole in the wall between the atria (upper chambers) of the heart. ASD is one of the more serious heart defects; it causes the clots from the veins to cross over from the right to the left side of the heart, whereupon they can pass into the arteries and result in a paradoxical embolism. If a clot is allowed to enter into arterial circulation, it can result in stroke. ASD also causes an increase in the blood flow to the lungs. The condition typically presents in childhood or adolescence. A large defect can result in congestive heart failure, while more minor cases of ASD can present as weariness, malaise, chronic respiratory infection, and failure to thrive. A close examination of the patient will reveal a fixed, split S2.

Diagnosis and treatment -- The risk of stroke that accompanies atrial septal defect means that even the most minor cases may require surgery. The diagnosis of ASD can be made after an echocardiogram indicates the characteristic blood flow from the right to the left ventricle, as well as a dilated right ventricle. An ECG will reveal right-axis deviation, while a chest X-ray will indicate elevated levels of pulmonary vascular markings. Only the smallest ASDs are allowed to resolve spontaneously; otherwise, surgical closure should be performed. This procedure can prevent complications like arrhythmia and Eisenmenger's syndrome, in which the left to right shunt of blood leads to pulmonary hypertension.

Patent ductus arteriosus

<u>Introduction and symptoms</u> -- A patent ductus arteriosus (PDA) is the failure of the vessel through which blood is shunted from the lungs before birth to close. Typically, a patent ductus arteriosus will close soon after birth, but if it does not then there may be a left to right shunt from the aorta to the pulmonary artery. Individuals are considered to be at a greater risk of PDA if they live at a high altitude or if their mother had a rubella infection in the first trimester. This condition is especially common in premature infants. Though it is often asymptomatic, PDA may present with chronic respiratory infection, congestive heart failure, and general failure to thrive. A close examination will display wide pulse pressure and a loud S2.

<u>Diagnosis and treatment</u> -- The diagnosis of patent ductus arteriosus depends on a color flow Dopple that indicates the left to right shunt of blood from the aorta to the pulmonary artery. Severe PDAs may present with left atrial and left ventricular enlargement that can be seen on an echocardiogram. A chest X ray will often indicate cardiomegaly, and an electrocardiogram will frequently indicate left ventricular hypertrophy. Minor PDAs may be allowed to resolve spontaneously, or they can be ligated through surgery. If the PDA is not needed for survival, the patient can be given indomethacin; failing this, surgery will be necessary.

Tetralogy of Fallot

The tetralogy of Fallot is a group of four heart defects that present at birth. These are: ventricular septal defect; pulmonary stenosis; right ventricular hypertrophy; and an overriding aorta. Individuals are at a much greater risk of this birth defect if they have Down syndrome, cri-du-chat syndrome, or trisomies 13 and 18. This condition frequently presents during infancy with cyanosis (a bluish tinge to the skin caused by insufficient levels of oxygen), dyspnea, and rapid weariness. The hypoxemia associated with the condition can result in alterations in mental condition and a failure to thrive. A closer examination will often reveal a systolic ejection murmur or a right ventricular lift. In order to make an accurate diagnosis, echocardiography must be performed, and a chest X ray should indicate a heart shaped like a boot. The basic treatment for the tetralogy of Fallot is to administer PGE sub-1 in order to keep the patent ductus artery open.

Coarctation of the aorta

Coarctation of the aorta is a congenital constriction of the aorta that hinders the flow of blood below the coarctation and increases the blood pressure above. Males with Turner's syndrome are at a heightened risk of this condition. This condition frequently is asymptomatic, although congestive heart failure and high blood pressure may present over time. A close physical examination will indicate that the systolic blood pressure is higher in the upper extremities. There may also be wasting in the lower extremities caused by the diminished flow of blood. In order to accurately diagnose coarctation of the aorta, an ECG, echocardiograph, and color flow Doppler should be taken. Surgery can be delayed until the symptoms present. Upon presentation, however, it may be necessary to perform a balloon angioplasty

Cystic Fibrosis

Introduction and symptoms -- Cystic fibrosis is a common genetic disease that affects the exocrine glands. This disease, especially common among Caucasians, is characterized by the production of abnormal secretions, which cause mucus to build up in the pancreas and intestine. This can impede respiration. About half of those afflicted with CF will present with failure to thrive or hindered respiration. Patients may also present with chronic pulmonary infection, cyanosis, bronchiectasis, hemoptysis, and nasal polyposis. Infants may present with meconium ileus, an obstruction of the intestine caused by an insufficient amount of the digestive enzymes produced by the pancreas. Other possible symptoms of cystic fibrosis are abnormal glucose tolerance, malabsorption syndromes, and type 2 diabetes.

Diagnosis and symptoms -- The diagnosis of cystic fibrosis usually depends on a sweat chloride test, which indicates cystic fibrosis if it is more than 80 mEq/L in adults and more than 60 mEq/L in children. Genetic testing can also help to provide evidence for a diagnosis of cystic fibrosis. If cystic fibrosis is not treated, it will prove fatal before the age of 5 for over 95% of those who have it. The treatment for the pulmonary manifestations of cystic fibrosis include chest physical therapy, anti-inflammatory agents, antibiotics, and DNase. Malabsorption can be remedied with pancreatic enzymes and fat-soluble vitamins A, D, E, and K. Physical therapy can be helpful in loosening the buildup of mucus in the lings and fighting infection.

Failure to thrive

The failure to thrive (FTT) is a child's inability to achieve the physical growth typical of his or her age. There is no official standard for failure to thrive, but most doctors consider it to be growth that is below the 3rd or 5th percentile for age, or growth rate that has declined precipitously. Some of the conditions associated with failure to thrive include poverty, low maternal age, chronic illness, HIV, and abnormal metabolism. Failure to thrive is considered to be organic when there is an associated medical condition, and inorganic when psychosocial factors are to blame. Infants who fail to thrive should be examined for systemic illness. In order to reverse this negative trend, a doctor may want to recommend supplementary feeding or hospitalize the child. Feeding may need to be performed intravenously.

Intussusception

Introduction and symptoms -- Intussusception is a condition in which one part of the intestine folds inside another. This generally occurs proximal to the ileolocal valve. This condition caused the supply of blood to that part of the intestine to be stymied, and so there may be intestinal obstruction. In extreme cases this can lead to the death of bowel tissue, and subsequent internal bleeding, perforation, abdominal infection, and shock. This condition most commonly affects children between the ages of 5 months and 1 year. The most common symptoms are sudden loud crying, often with the knees brought up to the chest. Other classic symptoms include vomiting and bloody stool. A palpation of the right upper quadrant may indicate a mass shaped like a sausage.

Diagnosis and treatment -- A diagnosis of intussusception must be made early on to prevent the adverse complications of the disease. An abdominal X ray and ultrasound may be performed in order to locate the obstruction. In order to positively identify the intestinal obstruction, however, the doctor needs to perform an air-contrast barium enema. This procedure can actually diminish the size of the obstruction and thereby effectively treat the condition; however, if it does not work then the patient may require a surgery to correct the intussusceptions and remove any dead tissue. Intravenous feeding and fluid can be continued until the patient has been able to perform a normal bowel movement. Therapy should also aim to correct any abnormalities in volume or electrolyte count.

Pyloric stenosis

Pyloric stenosis is a narrowing of the outgoing sphincter of the stomach, such that food is unable to pass easily into the duodenum. This condition most commonly affects first-born males and can cause feeding problems and projective vomiting. A close physical examination of a baby with pyloric stenosis will likely indicate a palpable epigastric mass shaped like an olive. There may also be visible gastric peristaltic waves. A positive diagnosis of pyloric stenosis can be made after an abdominal ultrasound indicates the narrow pylorus, and this is confirmed by a barium study. The patient should also be checked for hypochloremic, hypokalemic metaolic alkalosis. After managing whatever fluid or electrolyte imbalances the patient may have, a surgical correction with pyloromyotomy should be performed.

Bronchiolitis

Bronchiolitis is a disease in which the bronchioles (tiny branches of the air tubes within the lungs) become inflamed. This disease most commonly affects infants and children younger than 2 years, and is most often the result of respiratory syncytial virus. Individuals with bronchiolitis will typically present with slight fever, cough, apnea, and rhinorrhea. A closer physical examination will often indicate wheezing and tachypnea, as well as a hyperresonance when the chest is thumped. The condition can be positively diagnosed when an ELISA test of the nasal fluid reveals RSV, or when a chest X ray indicates overinflation of the lungs and atelectasis. If the condition is severe, then the patient should be hospitalized and given therapy for the symptoms. Hydration and oxygen are commonly employed to treat this condition.

Kawasaki disease

Kawasaki disease predominantly affects young children, and results in fever, conjunctivitis, and red and swollen lips and mucous membranes in the mouth. Children with Kawasaki disease may also present with cervical lymphadenopathy, maculoerythematous, and gingivitis. The diagnosis of subacute Kawasaki disease can be made after thrombocytosis and an elevated erythrocyte sedimentation rate are detected. Acute Kawasaki disease is diagnosed when the patient has a fever and four or more of the following: conjunctivitis; polymorphous rash; cervical lymphadenopathy; diffuse mucous membrane erythema; and erythema of the palms and soles. The treatment for this condition includes high doses of aspirin and corticosteroids. It is unknown at present whether Kawasaki disease stems from a virus or an environmental toxin.

Epiglottitis

Epiglottitis is a severe infection of the structures that cover the trachea during the swallowing process and forbid food from entering the lungs. This condition, if allowed to progress, can lead to fatal airway obstruction. Patients with epiglottitis may present with a sudden high fever, dysphagia, drooling, a muffled voice and a soft stridor. A patient will often unconsciously jut his or her chin forward in order to maximize air flow. The diagnosis of epiglottitis is usually based on clinical impression, though a lateral X-ray will indicate a swollen epiglottis that blocks the valleculae. Because of the serious nature of this condition, the patient should be immediately stabilized and taken to the operating room for an emergency endotracheal intubation or tracheostomy.

Croup

Croup is an infection of the larynx, trachea, and bronchial tubes that most commonly occurs in young children. This condition is usually caused by a virus, but occasionally it is a bacterial infection. The classic symptom of croup is a barking cough, though some patients may manifest fever, dyspnea, or a hoarse voice. The diagnosis of croup is usually made on clinical impression, although an AP neck film may be effective at illustrating the narrowing of the subglottis. Patients should be monitored closely at night, when breathing can become further disadvantaged by the supine position. Some patients may benefit from corticosteroids, though most cases can be resolved with fluids. In extremely severe cases, the patient should be given nebulized racemic epinephrine.

Apgar scoring system

The Apgar scoring set tells doctors whether there is a need for a newborn infant to be resuscitated. The five parameters of the test can be remembered by using the name of the test as a mnemonic, such that APGAR stands for appearance (color), pulse (heart rate), grimace (reflex irritability), activity (muscle tone), and respiratory effort. Each of these five areas is assigned a score from 0 to 2 at the one and five minute mark after birth. If the child scores from 0 to 3, then he or she needs to be resuscitated immediately; if the score is from 4 to 7, then the child may need to be resuscitated, and should be ventilated and observed; if the score is from 8 to 10, then the child has good cardiopulmonary adaptation.

Otitis media

Otitis media, otherwise known as middle ear infection, is typically caused by catarrh, flu, or pneumonia. Because children have a shorter Eustachian tube, which allows bacteria to enter more easily, they develop otitis media much more often than adults. Children with otitis media will typically present with fever, hearing loss, and irritability. It is quite common for parents to note that the child has been playing or tugging on his or her ear frequently. A physical examination will likely indicate erythema, bulging in the ear, and decreased movement in the tympanic membrane. It is possible that the tympanic membrane will even be perforated. The treatment for pediatric otitis media includes amoxicillin for ten days. Babies who feed from a bottle are more likely to contract this condition.

Neonatal jaundice

Introduction and subtypes -- Neonatal jaundice is typically due to the destruction of red blood cells; this process causes bilirubin to be released at a time when the liver is not yet ready to handle it and convert it into urine. An elevated serum bilirubin concentration is defined as more than 5 mg/dL. There are three major subtypes of jaundice: conjugated hyperbilirubinemia, which is always pathological; unconjugated hyperbilirubinemia, which can be either physiologic or pathologic; and kernicterus, which is a variation of unconjugated biluribinemia in which there is a permanent deposit of bilirubin made in the basal gangle, cerebellum, and pons. This last condition can be fatal, and may occur if the infant's level of jaundice exceeds 20 mg/dL.

Symptoms -- When examining a newborn for neonatal jaundice, a doctor should determine whether there is a possibility of intrauterine drug exposure, or if there is a family history of red blood cell defects or hemoglobinopathies. In this same line, it is important to determine whether the child is fed from the breast or from a formula. Physical signs of jaundice will include abdominal swelling, light-colored stool, dark urine, and weight loss. The increasing amount of bilirubin concentration may result in a cephalopedal progression of symptoms. Conjugated hyperbilirubinemia appears as intrahepatic cholestasis, extrahepatic cholestasis, and ToRCHeS infections; unconjugated hyperbilirubinemia appears as hemolysis, elevated enterohepatic circulation, sepsis, and physiologic jaundice.

Diagnosis and treatment -- In order to accurately assess a case of neonatal jaundice, a doctor will need to be able to differentiate between physiologic and pathologic jaundice. Physiologic jaundice does not present until 72 hours after birth, and tends to resolve within one week in term infants and within two weeks in preterm infants. During physiologic jaundice, the infant's bilirubin will rise less than 5 mg/dL a day, and will peak somewhere below 15 mg/dL. In all, direct bilirubin will be less than 10% of the total. As for pathologic jaundice, it is typically present within the first 24 hours of like, and can persist longer than a week in term infants and longer than two weeks in preterm infants. During a bout of pathologic jaundice, the infant's bilirubin levels will elevate more than 0.5 mg/dL every hour, and will peak above 15 mg/dL. Direct bilirubin will account for more than 10% of the total.

In order to accurately diagnose neonatal jaundice, a doctor must obtain a complete blood count with peripheral blood smear, Coombs' test, and estimates of the child's bilirubin levels. In suspected cases of hyperbilirubinemia, liver function, blood culture, bile acid, sweat, and aminoacidopathy/ alpha-antitrypsin tests should be performed. If a jaundiced newborn also has a fever, hypotension, and/or tachypnea, then the doctor should perform a full sepsis workup and should monitor the child in the intensive care unit. The treatment for neonatal jaundice should focus on the underlying causes of the condition; unconjugated hyperbilrubinemia can be treated with phototherapy if the bilirubin levels are only slightly raised, and with exchange transfusion if the levels are extremely high.

Respiratory distress syndrome

Introduction and symptoms -- Respiratory distress syndrome is when a sudden increase in the permeability of the barrier between the lung's capillaries and air sacs results in sudden respiratory failure. This condition predominantly affects premature infants. In technical language, the surfactant deficiency leads to poor lung function and atelectasis. Individuals are more susceptible to RSD if they have maternal diabetes, are male, and are the second born of a pair of twins. RSD typically presents in the first two or three days of life, as the child's respiratory rate raises above 60 per minute. The infant will also present with hypoxemia, cyanosis, grunting on expiration, nasal flaring, and intercostals retractions.

Diagnosis and treatment -- In order to exclude the possibility of infection, a doctor should measure the infant's arterial blood gas, and take a complete blood count and blood culture. A chest X ray is the most conclusive way of diagnosing RDS. If the infant does indeed have respiratory distress syndrome, then the X-ray will indicate bilateral diffuse alectasis, leading to air bronchiograms and a characteristic appearance of ground glass. If, instead, the child has transient tachypnea, the X ray will indicate deposits of amniotic fluid, which appear as periholar streaking in the interlobular fissures. If the child is suffering from meconium aspiration, the X ray will indicate rough, abnormal infiltrates, overexpansion of the lungs, and pneumothoraces.

If a child is suffering from congenital pneumonia in addition to respiratory distress syndrome, then a chest X ray will indicate patchy infiltrates; subsequent Gram stain and a finding of neutropenia will support this diagnosis. The treatment for RDS may involve continuous positive airway pressure, in which the air passage is kept open through a steady stream of air delivered through the nose. The possibility of death that attends RDS can be diminished by the administration of artificial surfactants. When a pregnant woman appears to be in danger of preterm delivery, she should be given corticosteroids in order to guard against the possibility of RDS; after the child is born, his or her lungs should be monitored with assessments of the lecithin-sphingomyelin ratio and phosphatidylglycerol.

Cerebral palsy

Cerebral palsy is an abnormal quality of motor function that is acquired at an early age and is caused by a nonprogressive brain lesion. CP may be pyramidal, in which there is spastic paresis of one or more limbs; or extrapyramidal, in which the person is nonspastic. Individuals with cerebral palsy may present with learning difficulties, speech deficits, and seizures. The limbs that are affected by the disorder often display hyperreflexia, increased tone, and/or underdevelopment. The diagnosis of cerebral palsy is made based on clinical impression. Physical therapy and special braces may help the child develop better motor control, while diazepam, dantrolene, or baclofen can be used to minimize spasticity.

Neuroblastoma

Neuroblastoma is a kind of cancer that arises during childhood. It occurs either in the adrenal gland or in the part of the nervous system that interacts with the adrenal gland. An infant with neuroblastoma may present with Horner's syndrome, in which one of the eyelids drops as the eyeball on that side sinks into the face. This indicates that the cancer has spread to the area behind the eye. The patient may also display hypertension, a nontender abdominal mass, anemia, and failure to thrive. It is possible that the cancer can compress the spinal cord, resulting in paralysis. It is important that neuroblastoma be diagnosed as soon as possible. Prognosis is also improved if the lymph node has not yet become involved in the tumor. The condition can be diagnosed after an abdominal CT scan indicates elevated vanillylmandelic acid and homvanillic acid. Tumors may be excised, and chemotherapy be used to prevent the spread of tumors.

Febrile seizures

Febrile seizures, which occur frequently in infants and young children, are usually not that important. There is usually no evidence of intracranial infection. These seizures usually occur during the rapid onset of the fever, and may be categorized as either simple or complex. A simple seizure lasts less than 15 minutes and is generalized; a complex seizure lasts longer than 15 minutes, and has a particular focus. The treatment of febrile seizure should attempt first to determine the source of any infection. If the child shows signs of central nervous system infection, then he or she should be given a lumbar puncture. In cases where the seizures are atypical, the doctor should obtain electrolytes, serum glucose, urinalysis, complete blood count including differential, and blood cultures. The patient may be given antipyretic therapy as the underlying cause of the fever is treated.

Wilms' tumor

Wilms' tumor is a form of kidney cancer that occurs during childhood. This condition mostly occurs in children from 2 to 4 years, and is more likely to occur in those children with a family history, neurofibromatosis, and as part of the conglomeration known as WAGR syndrome (Wilms', Aniridia, Genitourinary abnormalities, and mental retardation). The classic symptoms of Wilms' syndrome are microscopic hematuria, fever, hypertension, and a nontender mass on the abdominal region or flank. The tumors of Wilms' disease are associated with the conditions of hemihypertrophy and aniridia. A positive diagnosis of Wilms' tumor can be made after an abdominal CT scan or ultrasound indicates a bulky mass within the kidney. The most common treatment for Wilms' tumor is transabdominal nephrectomy and postsurgical chemotherapy.

Skin and Subcutaneous Tissue Disorders

Acanthosis nigracans

Acanthosis nigracans is a velvety hyperpigmentation of the skin that is related to insulin resistance, endocrine disorders, obesity, drugs, and malignancy. This condition may be predictive of type 2 diabetes later in life. The etiology of the condition is unknown, but it may be related to the action of growth factors on the skin. The patient will present with dark, dirty-looking plaques found in the flexural areas and in conjunction with prominent skin lines. Treatment aims at resolving the underlying cause. Erythrasma is caused by Cornyebacterium minutissimum and is common among diabetics and those who live in warm climates. Patients will present with a slowly enlarging area of macular patch, especially in the flexor areas. This condition is not typically symptomatic. Treatment generally includes topical or oral erythromycin.

Bullous pemphigoid

Bullous pemphigoid is characterized by chronic blistering eruption on an inflamed base. This condition is especially common in patients more than 60 years in age. It is caused by autoantibodies to BP1 and BP2 that are found in the basement membrane of the skin. Patients with this condition will present with prodromal erythematous and popular lesions which can lead to large, pruritic bullae that are filled with serous fluid and may result in deep erosions and crusts when they collapse. This condition almost never includes the mucous membranes, but is usually seen on the upper arms and thighs. The diagnosis of bullous pemphigoid can be made when immunostaining indicates fluorescence at the dermal-epidermal junction. Treatment for the condition is steroids: topical if mild, and oral if severe.

Atopic dermatitis (eczema)

Atopic dermatitis is a relapsing inflammatory skin condition that is characterized by pruritis. If the patient scratches his or her skin repeatedly, lichenification may occur. The patient will often present with dry, scaly, itchy patches and plaques with excoriations of the flexural areas and neck. Most of the time, the condition will emerge when the patient is an infant. Triggers of atopic dermatitis (also known as eczema) include skin irritants, stress, airborne allergens, and, on occasion, foods. The condition is often associated with asthma and allergic rhinitis. Individuals with this condition are also at an increased risk of contracting impetigo and cellulitis, as well as a severe HSV-1 skin infection. Treatment for eczema may include mild soaps and emollients, topical tacrolimus, topical steroids, and PUVA phototherapy.

Contact dermatitis

Contact dermatitis is a skin condition that is created when the individual comes into contact with a substance to which he or she has previously been sensitized. Some of the more common agents of contact dermatitis are poison ivy, poison oak, nickel, cosmetics, and certain perfumes and deodorants. Patients will often present with pruritis and rash, though they may also have edema, fever, lymphadenopathy, and generalized malaise. Diagnosis can usually be made from clinical impression, though in some cases skin patch testing may be useful. As for treatment, mild cases can be resolved with cool compresses and/or oatmeal preparation, while severe cases may require the administration of systemic corticosteroids.

Pemphigus

Pemphigus is characterized by shallow, painful erosions/blisters on the epidermal and mucosal surfaces that are caused by autoantibodies against desmocollins and desmogleins in the epidermis. The most common form of pemphigus is pemphigus vulgaris. Patients will present with gradually-worsening shallow erosions on their mucous membranes. These tend to lead to skin problems, and any blisters that are ruptured by pressure or friction will cause shallow ulcerations. This condition typically occurs in individuals between 40 and 60 years of age. Pemphigus may be diagnosed when immunological staining of the skin biopsy indicates autoantibodies against epidermal intercellular material. Also, a biopsy may indicate acantholysis. Treatment for pemphigus consists of oral steroids, though severe cases may require plasmapheresis.

Erythema nodosum

Erythema nodosum is an inflammation of the subcutaneous fat that produces sensitive erythematous nodules, typically on the anterior tibial areas. The lesions associated with this condition result from hypersensitivity reactions caused by drugs, infections, IBD, rheumatic fever, or sarcoid. This condition is most commonly found in young women. Patients with this condition typically present with painful, erythematous bilateral pretibial nodules that do not have ulceration. These nodules rarely are found on the face, arms, and trunk. Malaise, arthralgias, and fever often come before such a rash. The diagnosis of erythema nodosum is usually made after an incisional wedge biopsy. A chest X ray, cultures, and a Gram stain of the lesion may be taken as well; the Gram stain will usually be negative, as the lesions associated with this condition are reactive. The treatment plan for patients with erythema nodosum is supportive in nature; the legs should be elevated and the patient should be given bed rest and potassium iodide.

Erythema multiform

Erythema multiform is an immune-mediated cutaneous disorder that is caused by drugs, infection, vaccinations, or malignancy. Patients with this disorder will present with a mild prodrome of malaise and myalgias, and they are likely to have lesions on their extremities. The lesions associated with erythema multiform typically cover less than ten percent of the body. The condition is diagnosed when the patient discloses a history of exposure to the causative agents, and a skin biopsy indicates perivascular lymphocytes and necrotic keratinocytes. Mild cases of erythema multiform can usually resolve themselves without treatment, so long as the inducing agent is discontinued. If the condition is due to HSV, the patient should be given acyclovir.

Psoriasis

Psoriasis is a cell-mediated inflammatory disorder that results in epidermal hyperproliferation. Patients suffering from this condition will present with deep plaques covered in silver and white scales and sharp borders on the extensor surfaces. These plaques are not usually pruritic. Psoriatic arthritis is manifested in pain, tenderness, and joint stiffness. The diagnosis of psoriasis can be made after a skin biopsy indicates a thickened epidermis with no granular cell layer and the preservation of the nuclei within a hyperkeratotic stratum corneum. Many patients will display minor microabscesses. Most patients will have high uric levels, high erythrocyte sedimentation rate, and mild anemia. Treatment for psoriasis consists of topical steroids or topical calcipotriol for mild or moderate cases, and phototherapy and immunosuppressants for severe or generalized disease.

Lichen planus

The skin condition called lichen planus is often known by the 4 Ps: polygonal, purple, pruritic, papules. This condition is an inflammatory dermatosis that involves the skin and the mucous membranes. The condition is generally caused by drugs and is associated with hepatitis C. Patients with the condition will present with flat purple papules that are covered with an overlying network of white lines, known as Wickham's striae. It is also common for victims of the condition to have reticulate white hyperkeratosis on the mucosal surfaces. Lichen planus may be diagnosed after a biopsy indicates inflammation with hyperkeratosis, an elevated granular level, and a bandlike mononuclear infiltrate in the superficial dermis. Doctors typically prescribe topical steroids and oral antihistamines to reduce the itch, though especially bad cases may require PUVA, oral retinoids, oral prednisone, and cyclosporine.

SJS and TEN

Introduction and symptoms -- Stevens-Johnson syndrome (SJS) and toxic epidermal necrolysis (TEN) are similar, life threatening conditions caused by drug-induced immunological reactions. SJS is when less than 10% of the body surface area endures epidermal separation, while TEN is when the epidermal separation occurs over thirty percent or more of the BSA. Patients with this condition will frequently present with flu-like prodrome, skin tenderness, and painful mouth lesions. Also, they are likely to have started a new drug in the past few weeks. The patient will also have a morbilloform rash that evolves into coalescing red macules and flaccid blisters with full-thickened epidermal loss. Patients will have a positive Nikolsky' sign, and may be in danger of perishing from sepsis from superimposed bacterial infections.

Diagnosis and treatment -- The diagnosis of Stevens-Johnson syndrome is made through a skin biopsy revealing perivascular mononuclear infiltrate containing some eosinophils in the papillary dermis. The skin biopsy will also show some degeneration of the basal layer; extremely bad cases of SJS may show the formation of subepidermal blisters. A TEN skin biopsy will indicate full-thickness, with eosiniphilic epidermal necrosis and cell-poor infiltrate with a predominance of macrophages and dendrocytes and a powerful immunoreactivity to

TNF-alpha. Treatment for both SJS and TEN depends on the early identification and elimination of the agents that are causing the reaction. Patients may be given intravenous immunoglobin or analgesia, and severe cases may need to be hospitalized in the burn ICU in order to prevent dangerous fluid or skin loss.

Sebborheic dermatitis

Sebborheic dermatitis is a chronic superficial inflammatory disorder that is believed to be a reaction to the yeast Pityrosporum. Patients with this condition will present with pruritis during the neonatal and postpubertal periods, and will have yellow erythematous patches and plaques on their scalp, ears, and face. If a very small child has a severe case of sebborheic dermatitis, the physician should suspect that the child has HIV. Treatment for this condition consists of 1% hydrocortisone and topical antifungals for the face, body, and the intertriginous areas. The scalp can be treated with medicated shampoos, especially those containing selenium sulfide or zinc pyrithione.

Vitiligo

Vitiligo is characterized by areas of acquired cutaneous depigmentation that are the result of a loss of melanocytes. This condition is frequently associated with autoimmune diseases. Patients with this condition will frequently present with irregular white patches of skin, as the pigment slowly fades. This condition runs in families, and seems to be more common in people with dark skin. About 30% of those who suffer from vitiligo also suffer from thyroid disease. A positive diagnosis of vitiligo can be made either after antimelanocyte antibodies are found, or a skin biopsy reveals an absence of epidermal melanocytes. Treatment for vitiligo generally includes artificial tanning creams, steroid/tretinoin creams, and sometimes phototherapy. The lesions associated with this condition often go away of their own accord.

Cellulitis/ folliculitis

Cellulitis and folliculitis are skin infections that are generally caused by streptococci or staphylococci. Cellulitis is an infection of the subcutaneous tissue, manifested in hot swollen lesions. Patients with this condition may also have fever or chills. Cellulitis is particularly common in patients who suffer from diabetes, intravenous drug use, venous stasis, and immunocompromised states. Folliculitis, on the other hand, is an infection of the hair follicles, and it most frequently occurs in the distribution of facial hair. A positive diagnosis of these skin conditions depends mainly on clinical impression, though a wound culture may be helpful. If it is suspected that the patient has bacteremia, then a blood culture should be acquired. Mild and moderate cases are treated with oral antibiotics, while more severe cases require hospitalization and intravenous antibiotics.

Acne vulgaris

Acne vulgaris is a skin condition in which the hair follicles are blocked by sebum and keratinous material. This leads to the formation of cysts, otherwise known as comedones.

These comedones contain lipophilic bacteria that break sebum down into free fatty acids, which in turn results in the rupture of the cysts and inflammatory foreign-body reactions. Patients with acne often will have experienced recent changes in their level of androgen. The condition is most common during puberty, and especially in males. Acne may also be caused by the drugs lithium, steroids, oral contraceptives, and androgens. Mild acne is typically treated with topical clindamycin or erythromycin, benzoyl peroxide, and topical retinoids. Moderate cases of acne also should be treated with oral antibiotics, and sever cases should receive oral isotretinoin.

Herpes simplex

Herpes simplex is a painful, recurrent vesicular eruption of the mucocutaneous surfaces that is caused by HSV infection. First degree outbreaks of herpes simplex are typically longer and more severe than recurrent eruptions. The onset of the eruptions is presaged by prodromal tingling, burning, and pain. The condition may also include lymphadenopathy, fever, discomfort, malaise, and edema of the involved tissue. All of the grouped vesicles will be seen on an erythematous base, while recurrent infections will be restricted to the mucocutaneous areas that are enervated by the involved nerve. A positive diagnosis can be made after multinucleated giant cells are visible on an Tzanck smear. Herpes simplex looks a great deal like varicella-zoster virus, and so a culture may be required for differentiation. Treatment includes acyclovir ointment to reduce the duration of the viral shedding and to prevent recurrence. Patients may also receive oral or intravenous acyclovir in order to reduce the severity and frequency of the outbreaks.

Fungal infections

The fungal infection known as pityriasis versicolor (also known as tinea versicolor) is caused by Malassezia furfur. This condition is characterized by minute, scaly, hyper or hypopigmented macules that often enlarge and coalesce. The lesions associated with this condition sometimes itch a bit, but are generally asymptomatic. A potassium hydroxide prep will indicate short, blunt hyphae and small spores; treatment includes topical antifungal agents and selenium sulfide shampoo. Tinea corpores/ capitis is another kind of fungal infection, occurring mainly on the body or scalp. The patient with this condition will present with pruritic, ring-shaped erythematous plaques. A potassium hydroxide prep will indicate hyphae. Treatment includes topical antifungal cream for tinea corporis, and oral antifungals for tinea capitis and tinea unguium.

Lice and scabies

Lice are parasites that can infect the scalp, body, or pubic area. Patients with this condition will typically present with pruritus, and the condition can be diagnosed after a microscopic exam of the hair shaft indicates the nits, which will fluoresce blue under a Wood's lamp. An infection of lice can be treated with a permethrin shampoo or cream. Also, potential sources of reinfection should be decontaminated. Scabies infections are cased by parasites that burrow into the skin in order to lay eggs. Scabies infections are typically found among people who live in dirty conditions. The condition tends to get worse at night and subsequent to a hot shower. Scabies infection can be diagnosed after scrapings of the lesions with an oil or potassium hydroxide indicates the presence of the mites. Patients are treated with 5% permethrin cream, and antihistamines may be prescribed for the pruritis. Reinfestation can be forestalled by decontamination of bedding and clothing.

Impetigo

Impetigo is a contagious and autoinoculable skin infection that is caused by staphylococci or streptococci. This condition is especially common in children. Patients with impetigo will typically present with pruritic facial lesions covered in a yellowish crust. These lesions are most commonly found on the face, neck, and extremities. The nonbullous form of impetigo is characterized by superficial pustules surrounded by erythema; the bullous form begins as tiny erythematous macules which lead to thin-walled vesicles or bullae on an erythematous base. Impetigo may be diagnosed after bacterial cultures have been taken to test for sensitivities. The lesions should be washed with a mild soap, and systemic antibiotics may be employed against staphylococci and streptococci. This condition is highly contagious.

Rashes

Chickenpox -- Chickenpox rash progresses from macules to papules to vesicles which eventually rupture and form a hard crust. It is not unusual for lesions in different parts of the body to be in different stages at the same time. Patients with chickenpox also often have a fever, and are at risk of bacterial superinfection of lesions.

Rocky Mountain spotted fever -- The rash associated with Rocky Mountain spotted fever first appears on the palms and the soles of the feet, but it quickly spreads to the trunk and the face. This condition is caused by a tick bite, and is commonly accompanied by high fever, chills, and headache.

Lyme disease -- Lyme disease is caused by tick bites as well, and leads to a rash with circular lesions with a central clearing, reminiscent of a bull's-eye. These lesions are typically found in the moist areas of the body where the tick is known to bite.

Measles -- Measles patients will often develop white spots on buccal mucosa, otherwise known as Koplik's spots. These will typically occur about three days after a high fever. Patients will also have maculopopular rashes that spread downward from the head.

Rubella -- Individuals suffering from rubella are likely to develop a maculopopular rash that spreads downward from the head.

Erythema infectiosum -- Individuals with erythema infectiosum, otherwise known as fifth disease, may develop a "slapped-cheek rash of confluent erythema over their cheeks, followed by a maculopopular rash on their truck and extremities one or two days later.

<u>Scarlet fever</u> -- Scarlet fever causes a rash on the trunk that feels like sandpaper. Individuals with this condition may also develop a strawberry tongue and a circumoral pallor.

Necrotizing fascitis

Necrotizing fascitis is an infection of skin and fascia that develops rapidly and may result in death if it is not treated immediately. It is caused by Group A streptococci, mixed aerobic-anaerobic bacteria, or Clostridium perfringens. Patients with this condition will present with pain and unexplained fever. People are more likely to contract necrotizing fascitis when they have peripheral vascular disease, surgery, or other reaches in the skin or mucosa. Necrotizing fascitis of the perineal region is known as Fournier's gangrene. The patient will experience swelling, tenderness, induration, and/or bullae that lead to brittle skin with discoloration. The infection can quickly spread to the fascia and cause shock and multiorgan failure. Necrotizing fascitis is diagnosed based on clinical impression, and is treated with surgery to remove the necrotic tissue from the fascia and antibiotic therapy.

Molluscum contagiosum

Molluscum contagiosum is a poxvirus infection that is typically found in young children and AIDS patients. Patients will present with discrete, dome-shaped papules between 2 and 5 mm in diameter. These papules often have central umbilication. When children suffer from the infection, the lesions are often found on the truck, extremities, and on the face. Adults are more likely to have lesions in the perianal and perigenital regions. Immunocompromise must be suspected if the lesions are found in any other areas. Unless they are irritated, these lesions will be basically asymptomatic. A positive diagnosis can be made after the contents of a papule are expressed and Giemsa or Wright's stain is applied. The doctor should examine for large inclusion or molluscum bodies. The lesions associated with the condition will typically resolve after a period of months or years. Otherwise, they can be treated with curettage, liquid nitrogen cryotherapy, or by the application of trichloroacetic acid.

Varicella zoster

When an individual has a first degree infection with varicella zoster virus, he or she will develop chickenpox. If there is a latent infection in the sensory dorsal root ganglia, this can reactivate and lead to herpes zoster or shingles. Patients with this condition are likely to be elderly or immunocompromised, and are the vesicular eruptions are likely to be preceded by fever, dyesthesias, malaise, and headache. Painful eruptions will then occur in a dermatormal distribution. The diagnosis of varicella zoster is usually made through clinical impression, but in uncertain cases a Tzanck smear may be helpful in looking for multinucleated giant cells. Treatment typically includes antivirals within 72 hours of the appearance of lesions.

Pityriasis rosea

Pityriasis rosea is a mild and self-limited subcutaneous eruption that is associated with HHV-6. It is usually seen in connection with children who suffer from pruritis. The condition is manifested in a diffuse eruption of round erythematous papules and plaques that are covered with a thin, papery white scale. The individual's trunk will likely have a pattern of pustules reminiscent of a Christmas tree, which is preceded by a solitary, smaller patch (known as a herald patch). Pityriasis rosea is diagnosed after it has been distinguished from second degree syphilis. The lesions themselves are self-limited and will resolve themselves, but pruritus may require special treatment.

Neurocutaneous syndromes

Tuberous sclerosis appears on the skin as thickened patches, ash leaf spots, and angiofibromas. Patients with this condition may also suffer from seizures, periventricular tubers, mental retardation, and kidney or heart disorders. Neurofibromatosis is characterized by beige spots, neurofibromas, and axillary freckling. Patients with this condition often also have Lisch nodules, optic nerve gliomas, renovascular hypertension, scoliosis, and seizures. Sturge-Weber syndrome is characterized by a dark burgundy stain on the face, as well as the presence of seizure, mental retardation, and visual impairment. Von-Hippel-Lindau syndrome is characterized by hemangiomas, though patients with this condition may also manifest retinal vascular hamartomas, renal cell cancer, and polycythemia.

Lichen sclerosus

Lichen sclerosus is a chronic but benign condition in which there is inflammation and epithelial thinning. This condition often affects the skin in the anogenital area, especially among postmenopausal women. This condition is often pruritic and painful. An examination will find white, confluent papules, macules, and plaquea. Lesions are often found on the truck, neck, and the oral mucosa. In very rare cases, there is a risk of developing squamous cell carcinoma. A skin biopsy will often indicate hyperkeratotic epidermis with follicular plugging, which progresses to atrophy. Treatment for this condition usually includes short-term, high-potency topical glucocortisteroids and/or oral hydrochloroquine.

Basal cell carcinoma

Basal cell carcinoma is the most prevalent form of skin cancer; it is most often found on the head and neck. Basal cell carcinoma often occurs after prolonged exposure to the sun. A positive diagnosis of basal cell carcinoma is made after a skin biopsy indicates basophilic cells that are palisading with retraction. Basal cell carcinoma does not usually metastasize, but it has been known to destroy normal tissue. There are five histological patterns of basal cell carcinoma: nodular, micronodular, infiltrative, superficial, and morpheaform. Treatment protocol will depend on the characteristics of the tumor, including its histologic type. Some of the treatment options are curettage, surgical excision, cryosurgery, and radiation therapy. The best way to guard against basal cell carcinoma is with UVA/UVB sunscreens and by avoiding excessive exposure to the sun.

Seborrheic keratosis

Seborrheic keratosis is a benign epithelial tumor that looks as if it had been placed on the skin. These tumors are typically brown, and are most commonly found on the face, trunk, and the upper extremities. This condition is often confused with melanoma. The difference is that while melanomas have a smooth surface with a varying elevation, color, and density, seborrheic keratoses will have a uniform appearance over their entire surface. Seborrheic keratoses do not require any treatment after they are diagnosed. If a number of these keratoses erupt acutely at about the same time, this is known as the sign of Lesar-Trelat, and is indicative of an underlying malignancy.

Squamous cell carcinoma

The risk factors associated with squamous cell carcinoma include exposure to the sun, ionizing radiation, actinic keratosis, immunosuppression, arsenic, and industrial carcinogens. Individuals suffering from this condition typically have gradually developing, asymptomatic exophytic nodules with varying degrees of scaling or crusting. These nodules are usually found on the scalp, the backs of the hands, and the superior face of the pinna. Positive diagnosis of squamous cell carcinoma can be made after a skin biopsy indicates irregular masses of anaplastic epidermal cells that are spreading all the way down to the dermis. Treatment for the condition typically includes surgical excision of the nodules, radiation, or Mohs' micrographic surgery. Squamous cell carcinoma can be prevented with UVA/UVB sunscreens and conscientious avoidance of prolonged exposure to the sun.

Actinic keratosis

Actinic keratosis is a premalignant lesion that is caused by exposure to the sun and is confined to the epidermis. This condition presents as asymptomatic, coarse papules that have poorly demarcated erythematous bases and areas of white, superficial scaling. This condition has the potential to progress to squamous cell carcinoma. The positive diagnosis of actinic keratosis can usually be made after a skin biopsy indicates areas of dysplastic squamous epithelium that have not yet penetrate the dermis. Treatment for the condition typically involves cryosurgery, topical 5-FU, curettage, or a chemical peel. The best way to avoid actinic keratosis is with UVA/UVB sunscreens.

Melanoma

Melanoma is a melanocytic malignancy that is associated with sun exposure, fair skin, family history, xeroderma pigmentosum, proliferation of nevi, and the presence of dysplastic nevi. Patients with this condition may present with a pigmented skin lesion that has recently changed in size or appearance. Melanoma is typically asymptomatic until it is well developed, though it is possible for it to present with pruritus and slight discomfort. Lesions from melanoma appear on the areas that have been exposed to the sun and on the plantar surface of the feet. Doctors may remember the general pattern of melanoma lesions with the mnemonic ABCD: asymmetric, borders irregular, color variegated, and diameter greater than

6 mm. Melanoma can be diagnosed after a skin biopsy indicates melanocytes with a large number of atypical cells, accompanied by melanocytic invasion into the dermis. The most common form of treatment is surgical excision. Lymph node dissection is required in cases where the depth of the nodule is particularly great. Metastatic disease must be treated with chemotherapy.

Kaposi's sarcoma and rosacea

Kaposi's sarcoma is caused by HHV-8, and is extremely common in AIDS patients. Patients with this condition are likely to present dark red, thin, round plaques on skin and mucosa. A positive diagnosis of Kaposi's sarcoma can be made after a skin biopsy indicates a proliferation of small vessels and narrow intercellular slits with extravasated red blood cells. Treatment includes antiretrovirals for HIV, and chemotherapy for the lesions.

Rosacea is a chronic disorder of the pilosebaceous units that involves increased reactivity of the capillaries to heat. This condition is especially common among fair-skinned females. Rosacea typically begins as small papules or pustules, erythema, and telangiectasias on the cheeks, chin, and forehead. Male victims may develop rhinopyma. Treatment for rosacea includes topical metronidazole, sulfur lotions, and oral tetracycline/isotretinoin.

Mycosis fungoides

Mycosis fungoides is a cutaneous T-cell lymphoma that has no known cause. It typically emerges as thin, scaly patches that successively evolve into plaques, nodules, and tumors. If the infiltration is excessive, it can cause the patient to develop a lion-like appearance. Mycosis fungoides often causes intractable pruritus. A positive diagnosis of the condition can be made after a skin biopsy indicates an infiltration of odd lymphocytes with convoluted cerebriform nuclei in the upper dermis, and microabscesses in the epidermis. These tiny abscesses are known as Pautrier's microabscesses. Also, immunostaining will indicate T rather than B cells. Treatment for this condition includes PUVA phototherapy, topical nitrogen mustard, total-body electron beam irradiation, as well as systemic and topical retinoids. Complications associated with the condition include Sezary's syndrome, sepsis, and the progression to high-grade lymphoma.

Malignant melanoma

A superficial spreading of malignant melanoma is typically dark brown, variegated, and has an irregular shape. This spreading most commonly occurs on the back and on the legs among individuals between the ages of 30 and 60, and is the most common type of malignant melanoma. Nodular melanoma is characterized by uniform, dark blue nodules that crop up quickly and are likely to occur in any part of the body. Acral-lentinginous melanoma is characterized by a marked variegation of brown or black macules and papules on the palms, soles of the feet, mucous membranes, and nails. This form of melanoma is most common in Asian and African-American males in their 60s. Finally, lentigo maligna melanoma is characterized by flat-topped, brown and black regions that appear on the head, neck, and any regions that are commonly exposed to the sun. Lentigo maligna melanoma is most common in fair-skinned individuals in their 60s.

Musculoskeletal & Connective Diseases

Spinal stenosis

Spinal stenosis is a narrowing of the spinal canal that is typically caused by the degeneration of the discs between the vertebrae; this problem can lead to a compression of the nerve roots. Patients suffering from spinal stenosis will typically present with neck or back pain or numbness, leg cramps, and will generally find that the symptoms improve when the hips are bent. A radiograph will typically show progressive degeneration in the spine and an MRI or CT scan will indicate spinal stenosis. The treatment protocol for mild spinal stenosis is NSAIDs and abdominal exercises; for advanced cases, epidural steroid injections can be effective; for refractory cases, a surgical laminectomy can be helpful in the short-term.

Herniated disk

A herniated disk is one that protrudes from between two vertebrae and presses on a nerve root. Herniated disks are responsible for sciatica, which is pain that radiates to the lower back, leg, and back of the knee. Herniated disks most commonly occur in the lumbar region. Patients with herniated disks will present with sudden lower back pain, paresthesia, muscle weakness, and atrophy or contractions. It is possible for large midline herniations to cause cauda equina syndrome, in which there is dull pain in the lower back and upper buttocks and possible disturbances of bowel and bladder function. Diagnosis of a herniated disk can be made based on clinical impression, though a doctor may want to obtain a plain radiograph if he or she suspects other causes of the back pain. Herniated disks tend to resolve themselves within about four weeks with the help of rest, heat, physical therapy, and NSAIDs.

Duchenne muscular dystrophy

Duchenne muscular dystrophy is a severe form of muscular dystrophy that predominantly affects boys and is often deadly. It is an x-linked recessive disorder that results from a deficient amount of dystrophin, a cytoskeletal protein. Patients with DMD will usually be between 3 and 5 years of age, and will present with increasing clumsiness, fatigability, balance problems, and difficulty walking on the toes. This last problem is the result of the shortening of the gastrocnemius. It is common for patients with DMD to also be mentally retarded. A positive diagnosis of DMD can be made after the patient tests negative on a dystrophin immunostain, and an electromyography indicates elevated recruitment as well as polyphasic potentials. If a muscle biopsy is taken, it will likely indicate degeneration and fibrosis. Physical therapy, possible accompanied by Achilles tendon release, is the most effective treatment for this condition.

Ankylosing spondylitis

Ankylosing spondilitis is chronic inflammation of the spine and the sacroiliac joints of the lower back. If it progresses very far, it can actually lead to a fusing of the joints. Males with a family history of ankylosing spondylitis are at a greater risk of developing the condition. Patients with this condition will typically present with lower back pain that becomes worse with inactivity and in the morning. It is also possible for the patient to develop anterior uveitis (an inflammation of the eye) or even third-degree heart block. In order to make an accurate diagnosis of ankylosing spondylitis, a doctor must rule out reactive arthritis and psoriatic arthritis. A positive diagnosis of ankylosing spondylitis can be made after the patient has a positive human leukocyte antigen-B27 score and a radiograph indicates the characteristic bamboo spine and fused sacroiliac joints. Treatment for this condition includes NSAIDs for painful symptoms and stretching calisthenics to improve posture and breathing. Individuals with refractory cases of ankylosing spondylitis should receive tumor necrosis factor inhibitors.

Gout

Introduction and symptoms -- Gout is a condition in which the afflicted individual has unnaturally elevated levels of uric acid in his or her blood, persistent joint inflammation, decreased kidney function, and deposits of hard lumps of uric acid around the joints. Obese males, especially those from the Pacific Islands, are at particular risk of contracting the gout. The joint pain associated with gout will arrive suddenly, and usually affects the first metatarsophalangeal joint as well as the midfoot. The afflicted joints will become swollen, tender, and erythematous. Individuals suffering from chronic gout may develop tophi, nodular masses of uric crystals that are most often found on the elbows, around the big toe, and on the fingers.

Diagnosis and treatment -- The easiest way to diagnose gout is to identify the characteristic crystals in the body fluids, tissues, and joints. An aspirate of joint fluid will indicate long, negatively birefringent crystals. Though some patients will maintain normal levels of uric acid during an attack of gout, many will have levels elevated above 7.5. As for treatment, the best way to treat gouty arthritis is by reducing the inflammation with cold compresses and rest. Acute attacks of gout can be treated with NSAIDs like indomethacin, and sometimes steroids. Those patients who are either in a refractory state or are known to be chronic overproducers of uric acid may be treated with allopurinol; patients who are chronic undersecreters may be given probenecid.

Fibromyalgia

Fibromyalgia is a connective tissue disorder that is characterized by chronic pain, stiffness, and heightened sensitivity in the muscles, tendons, and joints. There will not be any evident inflammation. This condition is particularly common in women between the ages of 30 and 50, and is frequently linked with depression, anxiety, and irritable bowel syndrome. Although there is no specific test for the diagnosis of fibromyalgia, patients will likely present with multiple tender points. Most of the time, doctors arrive at a diagnosis of fibromyalgia after eliminating all other possible causes of the symptoms. This condition is typically treated with antidepressants, stretching, heat application, and hydrotherapy.

Osteoarthritis

Osteoarthritis, also known as degenerative arthritis, is a kind of arthritis that is caused by the inflammation, degradation, and destruction of the cartilage of the joints. This is the most common form of arthritis. Individuals are at a greater risk of developing osteoarthritis when they have a family history of the condition, are obese, or have a personal history of joint trauma. Patients with osteoarthritis will typically present with crepitus, a crackling or grating sensation in the joints. Patients may also experience a diminished range of motion, and radiography will indicate narrowing of the joint spaces and the presence of subcondral bone cysts. Osteoarthritis is treated with physical therapy, NSAIDs, and weight reduction. If the case is extremely advanced, a doctor may consider joint replacement.

Rheumatoid arthritis

Introduction and symptoms -- Rheumatoid arthritis is an autoimmune disease that is characterized by the chronic inflammation of the joints. Rheumatoid arthritis is considered to be a systemic illness because it can afflict many different parts of the body at once. This condition can lead to synovial hypertrophy and pannus formation, as well as the gradual wearing away of nearby bones, tendons, and cartilage. Individuals are at a greater risk of developing rheumatoid arthritis if they are female, between the ages of 35 and 50, and have the human leukocyte antigen DR4. Rheumatoid arthritis typically presents as sudden stiffness in the morning, sometimes accompanied by fever, malaise, and fatigue. One occasional symptom of the condition is Baker's cysts, swelling in the space behind the knee.

Diagnosis and treatment -- Individuals suffering from rheumatoid arthritis will generally be found to have elevated rheumatoid factor, and often will have an increased erythrocyte sedimentation rate, as well. If an aspiration is made of the synovial fluid, this will indicate turbid fluid, diminished viscosity, and a dramatically increased white blood cell count. Radiography is another good way to diagnose and assess the progress of rheumatoid arthritis: individuals who have recently developed the condition will display moderate swelling of the soft tissues, while those who have battled the disease for a while will often display narrowing and erosion of the joint spaces. The treatment for rheumatoid arthritis includes NSAIDs accompanied by a class of medications known as disease-modifying anti-rheumatic drugs (DMARDs).

Polymyositis and dermatomyositis

Polymyositis is an inflammatory condition caused by the spontaneous invasion of the torso muscles by white blood cells. Individuals with polymyositis will present with symmetric proximal muscle weakness. A similar condition, called dermatomyositis, entails the chronic inflammation of a muscle; this condition manifests as a slightly elevated red rash. A blood test on an individual with one of these conditions is likely to indicate high levels of creatinine phosphokinase, as well as aldolase. An EMG will indicate fibrillation, and muscle biopsy will confirm that the muscle tissue is degenerating and dying. Patients with either of these conditions can be treated with high-dose corticosteroids for 4-6 weeks, possible accompanied by azathioprine and/or methotrexate.

Scleroderma

Scleroderma is a disease of the connective tissue that results in the formation of scar tissue in the skin and other organs of the body. Scleroderma most commonly manifests as the CREST syndrome: calcinosis, Reynaud's phenomenon, esophageal dysmotility, sclerodacytly, and telangiectasias. This is a limited form of the disease; there is also a diffuse form that affects a variety of internal and external areas. Individuals suffering from scleroderma will often present with a thickening of the skin, face, or distal extremities. A positive diagnosis of scleroderma can be made after rheumatoid factor and antinuclear antibody are found to be positive; in the case of CREST syndrome, the patient will also manifest with anticentromere antibodies. If the patient is found to have Anti-Scl-70 antibodies, he or she has a poor prognosis. The basic treatment protocol for scleroderma depends in part on the organs that are afflicted; steroids and penicillin are commonly prescribed for dermatological changes, while calcium channel blockers may be helpful in combating Reynaud's phenomenon.

Systemic lupus erythematous

Introduction and symptoms -- Systemic lupus erythematous is the form of lupus that involves the internal organs. This is an autoimmune disorder that is caused by an antibody-mediated cellular attack and the deposition of antigen-antibody complexes. Patients with SLE may have rather nonspecific symptoms. The basic diagnostic criteria of SLE have been organized by the acronym DOPAMINE RASH: discoid rash, oral ulcers, photosensitivity, arthritis, malar rash, immunologic criteria, neurological symptoms, elevated erythrocyte sedimentation rate, renal disease, antinuclear antibodies, serositis, and hematologic abnormalities. If a patient has four of these symptoms, then it is likely that he or she has systemic lupus erythematous.

Diagnosis and treatment -- The positive test for antinuclear antibodies is a strong indication of systemic lupus erythematous. It is also very suggestive of SLE when a patient has anti-dsDNA antibodies and anti-Sm antibodies. Cases of SLE that are drug-induced will always manifest with the presence of antihistone antibodies, though this presence does not specify that the individual is suffering from SLE. The treatment of SLE will be aimed at decreasing the level of inflammation and controlling the patient's level of autoimmune activity. One way for the patient to avoid episodes is by avoiding sun exposure and by maintaining medication faithfully. The mild joint symptoms of this condition are often treated with NSAIDs, while the more acute symptoms may require steroids. The psychiatric symptoms of SLE should be treated as necessary.

Temporal arteritis

Introduction and symptoms -- Temporal arteritis, also known as giant cell arteritis, is the inflammation of the walls of the arteries, in particular the carotid and aorta. One of the more serious possibilities associated with temporal arteritis is a blockage of the central retinal artery that can lead to blindness. Individuals are considered to be at a greater risk of temporal arteritis when they are above the age of 50, female, and suffer from polymylagia rheumatica. The typical symptoms of the condition are headache, a pain in the jaw after chewing, and a heightened sensitivity in the scalp, in particular over the inflamed arteries on either side of the head. Individuals with temporal arteritis may also present with fatigue, slight fever, and weight loss.

Diagnosis and treatment -- A diagnosis of temporal arteritis usually depends on the biopsy of an artery. The examining doctor should look for tell-tale thrombosis, a necrosis of the media, and any giant cells, lymphocytes, or plasma cells. A patient with temporal arteritis will also likely have an erythrocyte sedimentation rate that is greater than 75, and will indicate some level of diminished vision during an ophthalmologic evaluation. Temporal arteritis is typically treated with high doses of cortisone medications, especially prednisone. This drug therapy should continue for one or two months. Even after being weaned off of the medication, the patient should be monitored and given frequent eye exams.

Polymyalgia rheumatica

Polymyalgia rheumatica (PMR) is a disorder of the muscles and joints in which the person suffers from pain and stiffness on both sides of the body, and in particular in the shoulders, arms, neck, and buttocks. This condition predominantly affects women above the age of 50. Individuals suffering from PMR will often say that they have a hard time getting out of a chair. Other, less common symptoms include fever, malaise, and weight loss. A subsequent blood test will often reveal a dramatically elevated erythrocyte sedimentation rate, and possibly anemia. The most common treatment for polymyalgia rheumatica is a low dose of prednisone, typically between 10 and 20 mg a day.

Endocrine & Metabolic Disorders

Type 1 Diabetes Mellitus

Type I diabetes mellitus is caused by autoimmune pancreatic beta-cell destruction that leads to insulin deficiency and an irregular fuel metabolism. The most common symptoms of diabetes mellitus are polyuria, polydipsia, polyphagia, and rapid weight loss. It is also possible that patients may present with ketoacidosis. This condition is associated with human leukocyte antigen DR3 and DR4. In order to make a diagnosis of Type I diabetes, at least one of the following conditions must be met: the patient has a fasting plasma glucose level greater than or equal to 126 mg/dL on two different occasions; the patient has a random plasma glucose level greater than or equal to 200 mg/dL; or the patient has a 2-hour postprandial glucose level that is greater than or equal to 200 mg/dL after the administration of a glucose tolerance test on two different occasions. Treatment includes insulin; the patient is required to monitor his or her own insulin levels. The patient should also have routine hemoglobin A sub-1c, blood pressure, foot, dilated-eye, and annual microalbuminuria exams, and a lipid profile every couple of years.

Type 2 diabetes mellitus

Introduction and symptoms -- Type 2 diabetes mellitus is a dysfunction in glucose metabolism, in which the insulin levels vary too widely. Patients will usually have the symptoms of hyperglycemia, though if the disease has onset the symptoms may be more severe, and may include serious complications. Patients will likely have poor glycemic control and nonketonic glycemia. This form of diabetes is most common in obese adults, especially those with a genetic predisposition to the disease. A positive diagnosis of Type 2 diabetes mellitus can be made according to the same conditions as Type I diabetes. Every person should be tested for Type 2 diabetes at age 45 (and re-tested every three years), regardless of whether they have the risk factors. Individuals with an impaired fasting glucose should be tested even more frequently.

Diagnosis and treatment -- Individuals who are diagnosed with Type 2 diabetes mellitus should immediately adjust their diet and exercise regimens. The following oral medications may be prescribed: sulfornylurea, an insulin secretagogue which can cause hypolglycemia and weight gain; meglinitinides, which work are insulin secretagogues with a shorter duration; metformin, which inhibits hepatic gluconeogenesis but may increase the peripheral sensitivity to insulin and can lead to weight loss, upset stomach, and is not recommended for the elderly; thiazolidinediones, which increase sensitivity to insulin; and alpha-glucosidase inhibitors, which decrease the intestinal absorption of carbohydrates. Insulins and statins are also important parts of the treatment regimen. Finally, patients with Type 2 diabetes have to keep track of their blood pressure.

Complications of diabetes mellitus

One chronic complication of diabetes mellitus is retinopathy, which appears only after diabetes has been extant for at least three years. This can be prevented with annual eye exams and laser photocoagulation therapy for retinal neovascularization. Another complication is diabetic nephropathy, which is characterized by microalbuminuria preceded by glomerular hyperfiltration. Still another is neuropathy, in which the patient has foot pain, infections, and diabetic ulcers. This condition can be avoided with foot care and analgesics. Finally, some diabetics may develop macrovascular complications, which may be cardiovascular, cerebrovascular, or peripheral in nature. The number one cause of death among diabetics is cardiovascular disease.

One of the complications of treatment for diabetes mellitus is the so-called Dawn phenomenon, in which the diminished effectiveness of insulin in the early morning leads to hypoglycemia. One of the acute complications of DM treatment is diabetic ketoacidosis, in which stress or failure to follow an insulin regimen leads to a hypoglycemic crisis. Patients in this condition may have abdominal pain, Kussmaul respirations, and a fruity breath odor. They should be given fluids, potassium, and insulin. Another acute complication is nonketotic hyperglycemia, in which the patient becomes extremely dehydrated and may experience mental status changes. This condition only occurs in individuals with Type 2 diabetes.

Tests for thyroid function

There are a few common tests of thyroid function. A radioactive iodine uptake and scan measures the amount of iodine that is taken up by the thyroid. A total T sub-4 measurement is mostly effective, but because levels can be altered by disorders of the binding proteins it is not considered to be conclusive. A T sub-3 resin uptake can help correct the errors made by a total T sub-4. A free T sub-4 measurement is the most commonly used screening test for measuring the levels of thyroid hormones. The best test for measuring the function of the thyroid, however, is the thyroid-stimulating hormone measurement; if an individual has high TSH, then he or she may have first degree hypothyroidism, while if levels are low then the individual may have first degree hyperthyroidism.

Metabolic syndrome

Metabolic syndrome is also known as Syndrome X, or insulin resistance syndrome. Patients who have this condition are more likely to develop coronary artery disease or to perish from a cardiovascular event. They are likely to present with abdominal obesity, high blood pressure, impaired glycemic control, and dyslipidemia. In order to receive a positive diagnosis of metabolic syndrome, a patient must meet three of the following criteria: abdominal obesity; triglyceride levels greater than or equal to 150 mg/dL; HDL cholesterol less than 40 mg/dL for men and less than 50 mg/dL for women; blood pressure greater than or equal to 130/85; and a fasting glucose level greater than or equal to 110 mg/dL. Treatment for this condition must include immediate and rapid weight loss, rapid lowering of cholesterol, and strict control of blood pressure.

Hypothyroidism

The most common cause of hypothyroidism is Hashimoto's thyroiditis. Patients that have hypothyroidism along with decreased mental function, hypothermia, and other symptoms are said to be in a myxedema coma. Patients with this condition will present with weakness, fatigue, intolerance to cold, constipation, weight gain, depression, irregularities in menstruation, and hoarseness. A positive diagnosis can be made after tests indicate elevated thyroid-stimulating hormone levels and diminished T sub-3 and sub-4 levels. Patients diagnosed with uncomplicated hypothyroidism should be given levothyroxine; those with subacute thyroiditis should be given NSAIDs or oral steroids; and patients with myxedema coma should be given intravenous levothyroxine and hydrocortisone.

Hyperthyroidism

Hyperthyroidism is the condition which results in thyrotoxicotic conditions, like Graves' disease and toxic adenomas, in which the thyroid overproduces thyroid hormone. Patients with hyperthyroidism will present with weight loss despite increased appetite, intolerance to heat, anxiety, heart palpitations, more frequent bowel movements, insomnia, and, among females, abnormalities in menstruation. The condition can be diagnosed after tests reveal decreased thyroid-stimulating hormone, and increases in T sub-3 and sub-4. The treatment for hyperthyroidism traditionally involves three things: radioactive 131-I thyroid ablation, thyroidectomy, and antithyroid drugs. Some patients may be given propranolol for beta-adrenergic symptoms until the hyperthyroidism is resolved.

Thyroid neoplasms

It is not uncommon for an individual to develop mostly benign thyroid nodules, particularly as he or she advances in age. These nodules are usually asymptomatic upon their first presentation, though if the patient has a history of neck irradiation, cold nodules, and quickly growing nodules accompanied by hoarseness, then the patient has an increased risk of malignancy. If the patient has carcinoma, they will likely be palpable, firm, fixed, and nontender. The diagnosis of thyroid neoplasms can be made after thyroid-stimulating hormone and thyroid function exams. The most effective way to tell whether a nodule is malignant is fine-needle aspiration. Benign neoplasms simply need to be examined and given an ultrasound; malignant neoplasms require surgical resection; and in the case of an indeterminate neoplasm, a lobectomy should be performed.

Thyroiditis

Thyroiditis is an inflammation of the thyroid gland, and may be subacute granulotamous, radiation, lymphocytic, postpartum, and drug-induced. Patients will typically present with a tender thyroid, malaise, and upper respiratory infection if they have subacute or radiation thyroiditis. A positive diagnosis can be made after tests indicate thyroid dysfunction. This usually consists of hyperthyroidism followed by hypothyroidism, and a radioactive iodine uptake and scan should indicate consistently low uptake. Treatment may include beta-blockers for hyperthyroidism and levothyroxine for hypothyroidism. Patients with subacute thyroiditis should be given anti-inflammatory medication.

Osteoporosis

Osteoporosis is a common metabolic bone disease that cases the afflicted individual to have low bone mass and disruptions in the bones' microarchitecture. Osteoporosis is usually asymptomatic, though patients may suffer hip fractures, vertebral compression fractures, and/or distal radius fractures after enduring only slight trauma. A person's risk of osteoporosis is increased by smoking, high caffeine intake, amenorrhea, and steroid use. A positive diagnosis of osteoporosis can be made after tests indicate increased markers of bone turnover, and X rays indicate global demineralization after more that 30% of the bone density is lost. Dual-energy X ray absorptiometry will indicate significant ostopenia. Osteoporosis can be treated with supplements of calcium and vitamin D.

Multiple endocrine neoplasia

The condition known as Multiple Endocrine Neoplasia (MEN) is common in individuals who have autosomal-dominance inheritance. There are three subtypes of MEN. Type I, also known as Wermer's syndrome, causes pancreatic, parathyroid, and pituitary tumors. Type II, which is also known as Sipple's syndrome, is blamed for medullary carcinoma of the thyroid, pheochromocytoma, and parathyroid gland hyperplasia. Finally Type III, which used to be known as MEN IIB, is associated with medullary carcinoma of the thyroid, pheochromocytoma, oral and intestinal ganglioneuromatosis, and marfanoid habitus. The most commonly afflicted areas associated with the three successive kinds of MEN can be remembered by thinking of the "P" organs: pancreas (I), pituitary (II), and parathyroid (III).

Hyperparathyroidism

The majority of cases of hyperparathyroidism are caused by a single adenoma, while some other may be caused by parathyroid hyperplasia. Although most cases of hyperparathyroidism are asymptomatic, some patients may present with stones, bone pain, myalgias, abdominal pain, nausea, fatigue, depression, anxiety, or disturbances in sleep. A positive diagnosis of hyperparathyroidism can be made after the patient demonstrates hypercalcemia, hypophosphatemia, and hypercalciuria. If the condition is symptomatic, a parathyroidectomy may be recommended. If the patient is suffering from acute hypercalcemia, then he or she should be given intravenous fluids, intravenous bisphosphonate, and calcitonin.

Paget's disease

Individuals who suffer from Paget's disease have an increased rate of bone turnover. This leads to greater than normal resorption and excessive formation of bone. A mosaic-like pattern of lamellar bone should be evident. Though the exact etiology of Paget's disease is unclear, it is suspected to derive from viral infection and/or genetic predisposition. The condition is usually asymptomatic, but the patient may present with aching bones and joints, headaches, skull deformity, or nerve entrapment that leads to a loss of hearing. A positive diagnosis can be made after radiography indicates classic changes in bone, and laboratory tests indicate elevated serum alkaline phosphatase with normal levels of calcium and phosphate. Most patients are asymptomatic, however, and will require no treatment.

Acromegaly

Acromegaly is a condition affecting adults in which there is a benign pituitary growth hormone adenoma. Patients with acromegaly may present with coarsening of the facial features and enlargement of the jaw, hands and feet. Also, patients may have carpal tunnel syndrome, hypertension, arthritis, and bitemporal hemianopsia due to compression of the optic chiasm by a pituitary adenoma. A positive diagnosis of acromegaly can be made after an MRI of the pituitary indicates sellar lesions; the diagnosis is supported but not confirmed by elevated serum GH levels. Levels of insulin-like growth factor I will also be elevated. Treatment for acromegaly includes transphenoidal surgical resection or irradiative ablation of the tumor; the symptoms of refractory cases can be managed with the medications octreotide, pergolide, and pegvisomant.

Cushing's syndrome

Cushing's syndrome is most often due to the hypersecretion of ACTH from a pituitary adenoma. These adenomae are known either as Cushing's disease or central hypercortisolism. Some of the other causes of Cushing's syndrome include ectopic ACTH secretion from neoplasia, excess adrenal secretion of cortisol, and other iatrogenic factors. Patients will present with history of hypertension, central obesity, muscle wasting, thin skin with purple striae, hirustism, moon facies, and so-called "buffalo hump." They will likely present with depression, growth retardation, excessive hair growth, and symptoms of diabetes. A positive diagnosis can be made after a 24-hour free urine cortisol/ low-dose dexamethasone suppression test indicates morning cortisol is elevated after being suppressed the night before. Surgical resection of the hypersecretory source may be necessary, as may pituitary radiotherapy.

Adrenal insufficiency

First degree adrenal insufficiency is typically caused by autoimmune adrenal cortical destruction, otherwise known as Addison's disease. This will result in deficiencies of mineralocorticoids and glucocorticoids. A polyglandular autoimmune syndrome may include autoimmune destruction. Second degree adrenal insufficiency is caused by diminished ACTH production in the pituitary gland, which is generally caused by a sudden halt to the treatment of chronic glucocorticoids. Most of the symptoms for these conditions are nonspecific, though many patients will experience weight loss due to anorexia, weakness, and fatigue. Patients with Addison's disease are likely to display hyperpigmentation due to increased secretion of ACTH.

A positive diagnosis of adrenal insufficiency can be made after hyponatremia and eosinophilia are indicated. First degree adrenal insufficiency is specifically indicated by hyperkalemia. The diagnosis can be confirmed by measuring the plasma cortisol levels. If an individual has low plasma cortisol levels during a period of high physiological stress, then this confirms the diagnosis. Low levels are defined in this case as less than 20 micrograms/dL. The diagnosis can be excluded by a random plasma cortisol level of more than 20 micrograms/dL. Patients with adrenal insufficiency should be given glucocorticoid replacement treatment, with supplementary mineralocorticoid replacement if they have first degree adrenal insufficiency.

Hyperaldosteronism

Hyperaldosteronism is a condition caused by the over-secretion of aldosterone in the zona glomerulosa region of the adrenal cortex. This condition is usually due to a unilateral adrenal adenoma, though it can be caused by adrenocortical hyperplasia. Patients with this condition will typically present with hypertension, headache, polyuria, and muscle weakness. Individuals with severe cases may present with peripheral edema. Diagnosis can be made after the patient is found to have hypokalemia, mild hypernatremia, metabolic alkalosis, low plasma resin, and elevated 24-hour urine aldosterone. Treatment for hyperaldosteronism usually includes spironolactone for bilateral hyperplasia and a laparoscopic or open adrenalectomy of adrenal tumors.

Pheochromocytoma

Pheochromocytoma are chromaffin tissue tumors that are found in either the adrenal medulla or the extra-adrenal sites that secrete catecholamines; in other words, these tumors imitate the activation of the sympathetic nervous system. This condition is associated with von Hippel-Landau syndrome, neurofibromatosis, or MEN II/III syndromes. The patient will typically present with intermittent tachycardia, palpitations, chest pain, hypertension, headache, diaphoresis, anxiety, or tremors. A positive diagnosis of pheochromocytoma can be made after a CT or an MRI indicates a suprarenal mass. The usual treatment program for the condition is surgical resection. Before this procedure is performed, however, the patient should receive an alpha-adrenergic blockade in order to reduce the risk of intraoperative hypertension.

Congenital adrenal hyperplasia

Congenital adrenal hyperplasia is a category of inherited disorders that all stem from a deficiency of cortisol. The majority of cases of congenital adrenal hyperplasia are caused by 21-hydroxylase deficiency, which leads to diminished cortisol production. Female infants with this condition may have ambiguous genitalia, and males may undergo macrogenitosomia. The condition can be diagnosed after blood and urine checks reveal high levels of cortisol precursors and androgens. Treatment typically includes cortisol administration in order to decrease the levels of ACTH and adrenal androgens. As for surgery, this is only necessary when female infants are born with ambiguous genitalia.

Special Report: Additional Bonus Material

Due to our efforts to try to keep this book to a manageable length, we've created a link that will give you access to all of your additional bonus material.

Please visit http://www.mo-media.com/usmle/bonuses to access the information.